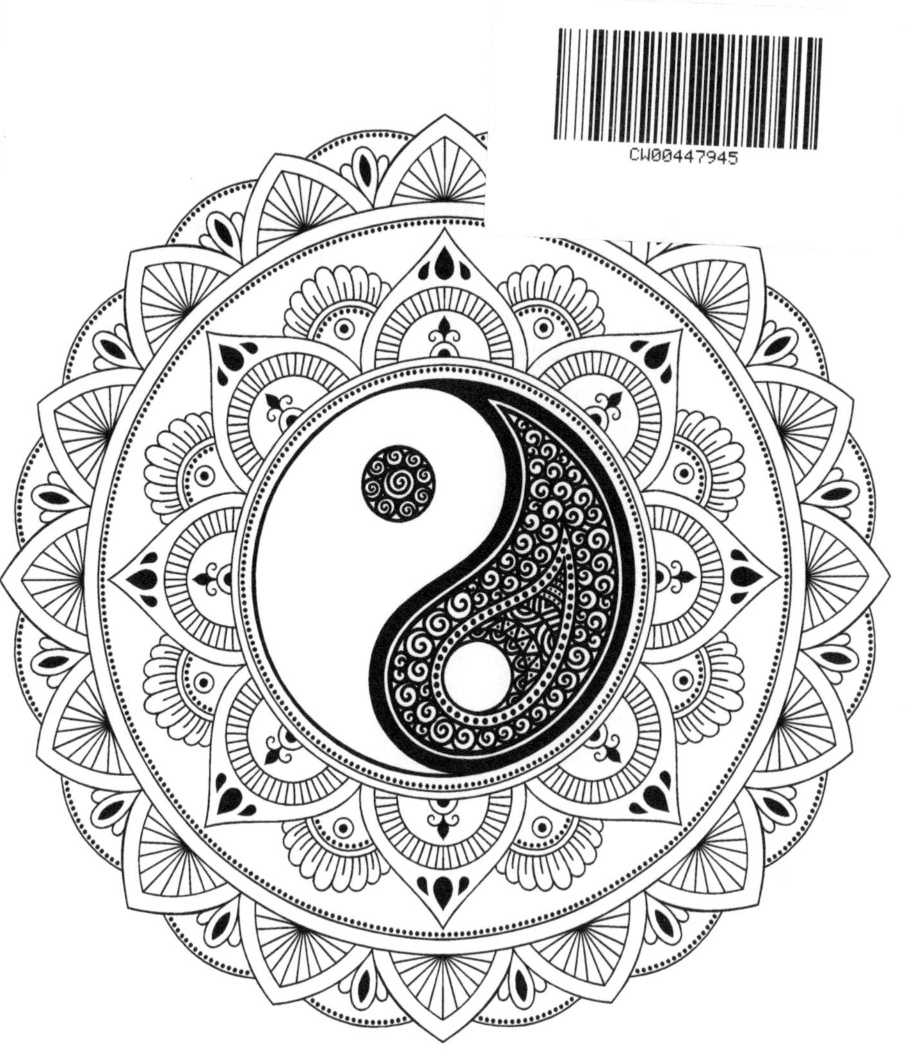

YIN MAGIC

How to be Still

SARAH ROBINSON

Published by Womancraft Publishing, 2020
www.womancraftpublishing.com

ISBN 978-1-910559-61-1
Yin Magic is also available in ebook format: ISBN 978-1-910559-60-4

Cover design, interior design and typesetting: Patrick Treacy, lucentword.com
Cover image © Hannah Dansie, hannah-dansie.com
Yoga sequence images: falconnadix and Baleika Tamara/Shutterstock.com
Mandala image: Katika/Shutterstock.com
Body Meridian image: Peter Hermes Furian/ Shutterstock.com

Womancraft Publishing is committed to sharing powerful new women's voices, through a collaborative publishing process. We are proud to midwife this work, however the story, the experiences and the words are the author's alone. A percentage of Womancraft Publishing profits are invested back into the environment reforesting the tropics (via TreeSisters) and forward into the community.

Medical disclaimer

The information provided in this book and other materials online are for reference and not a substitute for medical advice or direct guidance of a qualified yoga instructor.

Please practice with care and compassion for yourself. The author and publishers assume no responsibility or liability for any injuries or losses that may result from practicing yoga or witchcraft.

Not all yoga poses are suitable for everyone. Practicing under the direct supervision and guidance of a qualified instructor can help determine what poses are suitable for you. Always, if in any doubt, consult with your healthcare provider before practicing yoga or any other exercise program.

Also by Sarah Robinson

Yoga for Witches
The Yoga Witch Cook Book (eBook)
The Yoga Witch Cook Book: Yule Edition (eBook)

Acknowledgements

Thank you to Leilani Lea and to fellow Womancraft author Gina Martin, both certified acupuncturists and goddesses of wisdom, for helping me find my way amongst the medicine and meridians. As always, infinite gratitude to Lucy Pearce, for her tireless work whipping my muddled manuscripts into shape. And to fellow yoga witches Trish and Michelle for sharing their thoughts on the magic of yin!

Praise for
Yin Magic

Like a long, deep, beatific exhale, this gentlest book envelops you from the opening page – as soft as it is powerful, as accepting as it is radical – a treatise, toolkit and treasure, for all women who seek to re-member their nature.

Emine Kali Rushton, editor of *oh* magazine, poetess and holistic practitioner

Another beautiful and instructive book for these weird modern times from Sarah Robinson. A delight to read, Sarah is now a trusted resource in my empowering library.

Alice B. Grist, author of *Dirty & Divine* and *The Book of Tarot*

Sarah Robinson has a special talent for taking disparate and complex ancient systems and making them, not only accessible , but making their similarities so glaringly obvious that you wonder why you didn't see them before.

Sarah has drawn a path that helps the reader find these delicious connections and see the rich similarities and illustrative differences between Yoga and Chinese Medical theory. I learned a lot with this book and enjoyed every minute.

Gina Martin, Classical Chinese Medicine practitioner, M.S., Dipl. Ac. (NCCAOM), L.Ac., L.M.T., author of *Sisters of the Solstice Moon* and *Walking the Threads of Time (Books I and II of the When She Wakes series)*

Yin Magic is exactly what the world needs right now. An invitation to slow down; the reasons why it's essential we do that, as well as detailed guidance on how we do it. Engaging and fascinating, Yin Magic is an antidote to the world's default stress state. Robinson is also genius at breaking down in-depth philosophies and practices such as Tao, Yoga, Buddhism, Ayurveda, and Chinese medicine in a way that makes them relatable and applicable in our lives today.

Tamara Pitelen, author, energy healer and yoga instructor

CONTENTS

1

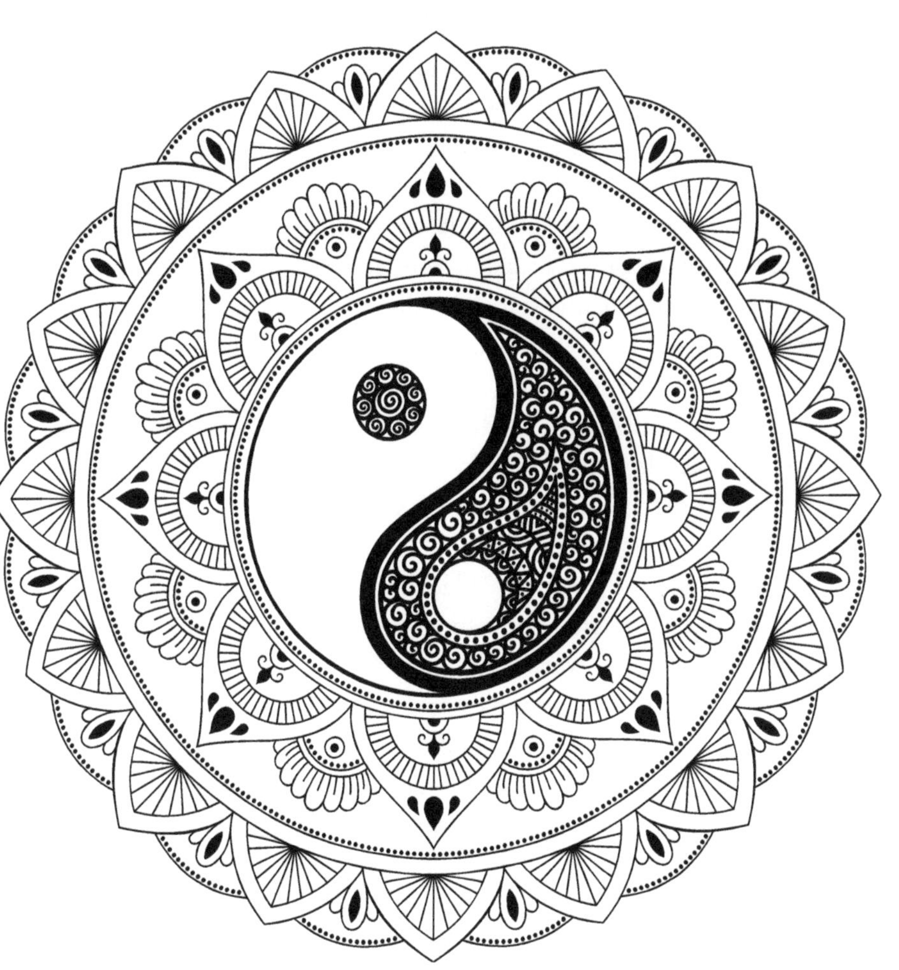

YINTRODUCTION

As a yoga teacher, I get the privilege of spending time with so many lovely humans. And over the years, I have noticed a pattern: most of us seem to struggle with being still.

As a woman living in the modern world, I recognise these struggles in myself, in my daily life.

As someone with a scientific background, I am intrigued by these patterns as evidence of an underlying issue, bigger than any individual. And so, I wanted to begin our time together by sharing a few stories, without judgment or criticism to the best of my ability, as living examples of what I observe.

I teach a regular class on Mondays at a local yoga studio. This yoga studio has two rooms – I teach in one, and at the same time, another teacher takes a dynamic class next door. It's a hugely popular class, and the teacher is excellent. In contrast; my yin yoga class is a very easeful start to the week, just as I like it: Monday as our Moon Day. One Monday in spring, two women arrived at the studio keen to practice yoga, but the dynamic class was fully booked. The receptionist said they were welcome to take my class, and they asked me what kind of yoga it was. As I told them, one of the women visibly grimaced and said "oooh no!" I laughed and then they laughed. And then they left. Preferring not to practice yoga at all that morning, rather than take a slow class.

I used to work at a university and went to the same on-site yoga class as my boss. She was the kind of person that you might describe as 'living on her nerves' – flighty and easily stressed. And without fail every hour-long yoga class we did, she would leave before the four-minute meditation at the end. In the two or three years we both went to this class she never stayed once for meditation.

I met a lady in a coffee shop who was new to town, we got talking, and she was also a yoga teacher. I invited her to join me for a yoga class the day after – as we were both free and a friend of mine held the class. I suggested we could have coffee and cake afterwards to give her a chance to meet another new person and fellow yogi. When I arrived at that class the next day, the lady and my teacher friend were already in the studio. And our new lady was not happy. "You didn't tell me it was a beginners' class," she said. My new friend was adamant that she, as a seasoned yogi, could not do a beginner class, so left. We never had our coffee and cake.

And I know why these stories stay with me: because I have been, and often still am, doing exactly the same thing! They jar in my mind because these behaviours reflect my own.

I so often speak of the joy of slowing down, only to spend weeks doing exactly the opposite.

Every retreat I run with my fellow yogis, I try to attend one of their classes. I successfully manage to never keep my mind on my practice, instead thinking about what we are serving for lunch, what sessions we'll do in the afternoon, if I have time for a shower before the next class... basically everything except the practice in front of me!

In a studio in Boston, I chose to do a handstand workshop over one on self-love.[i] In meditations I often start making shopping lists in my head.

A beautiful fellow yoga teacher I know rises every day at 5am to practice an hour or more of ashtanga (a dynamic style) yoga. I, conversely, flop out of bed into my dressing gown and into a Child's Pose. Ten minutes later I get up and say "That'll do!" and go make a cup of coffee. That's honestly what my practice looks like most days (sometimes there's more yoga, and some days it's just the coffee!). I joke with my lovely yoga pal about our contrasting morning routines. But I know full well those jokes are based in my own insecurity – I feel inferior to her and her dedicated practice. Obviously, this is silly, our practices are just very different. But it can be hard when people around us are seemingly achieving great things, we often feel that we need to keep up in some way (or if you are like me, make self-deprecating jokes about it, to cover the fact that I feel 'less than').

i Funny story, I actually ended up in the wrong studio, the teacher started playing "Let's Get it On" by Marvin Gaye – and I thought, well this is strange! It turns out I was in the self-love class, by mistake! (or not, if you think the universe played a part). It was a really fun class with an awesome playlist!

Scared to be Still?

I always make it very clear in my yoga classes that my students are free to leave early if they need to or if they don't want to do *savasana* (Pose of Relaxation). Everyone is on their own path: they may need to be somewhere, or have other things going on. I always want my students to feel at ease enough to do what they need to do. But I do wonder (and worry) how often my students, despite all I have said through the classes I teach, feel that being still, slow or restful is somehow 'pointless' – which it's not, as we will discover here together. Our avoidance of stillness can be almost pathological, which is why I have come to theorise that some people – perhaps many of us – are *scared* of being still.

When I notice people that seem unable to be still, I recognise that they are a reflection of my own shadow self: that part of me that always feels unable to slow down, or guilty when I do. I'd like to explore this together in this space, without judgement. So that we can begin to get to the bottom of this fear or aversion that so many of us have of being still and slow.

I invite you now to begin that enquiry.

Do you find value in slowness, or do you struggle to slow down?

What is it about being still or taking things slowly that you resist?

Do you get bored easily?

Does it seem like a waste of time?

Are you scared to be still in case feelings such as grief, sadness or anxiety catch up with you?

Perhaps you can't rest knowing that the washing up/school run/timesheets need doing…? If so, you're far from alone.

The Pressure to Live Your Best Life

The rise of 'burnout' or 'overwhelm' is due to many factors. Technology and social media are major contributors; providing us with endless streams of images of enviable lives. We're often told that only those who get up every day at 4am are successful; that you can – and should – teach your body to operate on less sleep; that you need to work out harder at the gym, always be advancing your practice: be faster, be more productive, push through barriers... You get the idea.

This has even spilled out into 'wellbeing'. There is increasing expectation that we should be creating morning rituals, hitting the gym, taking advanced classes, making picture-perfect granola bowls, growing our own herbs, meditating, working on passion projects on the side and then creating sumptuous organic family suppers. We simply can't measure up or keep up with this pace. This pressure to be perfect is a chronic stressor and can leave us feeling fatigued, cynical and detached.

We cram our days so full of activities and technological stimulation that settling down in bed can be the first chance we have all day to collect our thoughts. So, all of a sudden, thinking, worrying and processing information all kick in when we want to go to sleep. Our sanity during the day and sleep at night are suffering when we can't find stillness or peacefulness on a regular basis.

In a culture that celebrates continual expansion: from houses to social circles to businesses and 'influence', success is rarely depicted as a life of abundant time – time to tend plants, sip tea, write, sleep or sit in the sun doing nothing. But as we all know, time is the one thing money cannot buy. So maybe we should savour it as a luxury in itself – sometimes filling time with adventures, sometimes with nothing – consciously choosing time, letting go of, as much as possible, that which doesn't spark joy or satisfaction in some way.

We have this ideal of living our 'best life'... but we are so bombarded with ideas of what our best life should *look* like, we may well have forgotten or got separated from what our own best life should *feel* like. Often that thing is something that doesn't look that impressive: a nap, a quiet walk, turning down an invitation to a party and curling up with a loved one. A chance to slow down and pause can – must – be part of our best life.

Learning to Do Nothing

As our world increases in pace, we can learn that there is power in pausing. There is much to be gained, not from rushing and racing and doing, but from taking a seat and observing, listening and regrouping. Taking time to make choices about how we engage with this fast-paced society and the high expectations we set upon ourselves can help.

It sounds simple enough, but as meditators will know, doing nothing and achieving mental stillness can be a real challenge. A fast-paced world makes moments of complete stillness hard to create, especially in our 'always on' culture (and devices) which can cause cognitive fatigue. The more ways we have to connect, make it all the harder to disconnect and unplug. And even when we take time out, we may still feel a background buzz of anxiety, or distraction that we should indeed be 'doing something'. To engage and settle in purposeful stillness is a skill that takes time and practice.

The challenge is to live life in balance. If doing nothing feels just too challenging, how about trying to do less? Cancel one engagement or task this week and use that time to consciously slow down.

We can still find it hard to believe that 'doing nothing' is, in fact, doing something vital. And so, we may need regular reminders (like this book) that we do not always have to make things complicated for ourselves, that we do not always have to push ourselves to our limits. Intellectually understanding the tangible, measurable benefits of relaxation is all the more critical in today's super-dynamic society.

In yoga as well as in life, resting is a real skill that can be learned. As the world speeds up, many people are exploring options to slow down. Because of this, yin, slow and restorative yoga classes are some of the most popular classes I teach. I often find that people enjoy getting the 'permission' to settle into calm and comfort: into their comfort zone. Within this place, the body can rest and recharge, giving the mind a chance to process thoughts and the body a chance to release the tensions it has gathered through the previous day, weeks or months.

Changing Systems

Are you always rushed, and rushing, with no time for what you love, for what matters most?

How many times do you wake up feeling just as weary as when you went to bed?

How frequently do you feel overworked or overwhelmed?

Our nervous system has two different functional states that we may know as stress (fight or flight) and calm (rest and digest). They are controlled by the sympathetic nervous system (SNS) and parasympathetic nervous system (PNS) respectively.

The SNS is vital for our immediate survival, it works quickly to mobilise us (think a boost of adrenaline, quickened heart rate): if a bear comes to eat us, our SNS kicks in to get us the hell out of the way or put up a good fight. But for our long-term survival it's the PNS that helps us digest our food, relax enough to rest and engage in activities vital to our wellbeing: bonding, sharing and creating.

When the body is in fight or flight mode and the SNS is activated, the body and mind have one goal: to get you out of this situation as quickly as possible. Stress helps you reach a deadline. The body is working overtime to get you through this period of stress and to the end. Not to do your best, most profound work, no, just to get it done, and get you out of this stress state. And many of us experience these kinds of days or periods of work where we are just trying to get through, survive, to get it done. But then along comes another stress state, and another: the body, mind and organs are just trying desperately to get us out of this stress state again and again.

In contrast to the SNS, our PNS is slower to kick in, it needs time to be activated, it's something we need to settle into. And as we release into the PNS, we can release deeply held tension in the body, allowing for renewal and vital healing on many levels, physiologically and emotionally.

So much is put on hold and/or compromised when you are in fight or flight mode. Your body and brain functions are optimal when you are calm. I can't emphasise this enough. You might not quite believe it yet, as we've so many contradictory voices in the form of culture, media and conditioning. Just hold it in your mind as we journey through this book and be open to some ideas that may help you let go of this cult of speed and stress.

Activating the PNS can decrease anxiety and stress, calming mind and body. A host of benefits occur when our bodies are relaxed: our muscles soften, our heart rate slows, blood pressure is reduced... and that's not all! When we are relaxed our brains work more optimally, our sight and hearing improve, we digest our food properly, and our immune systems strengthen. All these things are put on hold and/or compromised when we are in the fight or flight mode, as we run on the primal instincts and reflexes of the SNS. So, whilst relaxing is an activity that in itself can be pleasurable, the after-effects of taking time to relax also bring real benefits to the body and mind.

Just like yin and yang, the sympathetic and parasympathetic systems function in complement to each other. But the quick-to-action SNS is more likely to dominate on busy days, so we need to do what we can to support the activation of PNS. Your 'fight or flight' system may have been dominant for months, or even years. And, especially if your stresses are mental and emotional – you may have gotten into the habit of living in your head, bombarded by the noise and demands of the world. This separation of mind and body can pull us away from the felt knowledge of our bodies.

So, in resting, we are creating big change: from one state of being and system of functioning to another. We are rebuilding a connection to our intuition, our deep sense of knowing, which anxiety and stress (among other things) can pull us away from. To recover from daily stress (or more serious burnout or trauma) the repair system in our bodies needs to be dominant. As we practice allowing the body to relax, its relaxation response engages and strengthens.

Finding the Off Button

We definitely all know that we need rest for energy. Our bodies remind us. But ironically, the tireder you are, the harder it can be to rest. Resting isn't easy if you are feeling stressed. It can be hard to find the 'off' button, or have power over it. But it is essential. So listen to your body seriously when it tells you it's tired. And do everything within your power to answer its call.

However, often the voices outside us are louder than our body's calls for rest. Often the external agents in our lives care nothing for our body's exhaustion, and we can feel powerless to refuse their demands. Or we can find ourselves so immersed in what we feel we *should* be doing, we can struggle to find the time to do the things that bring us joy, or things that help us unfurl from the busyness of life.

While many of us have certain levels of choice, I appreciate that some of us cannot just decide to take a break or do not have it in our power to step away from a really stressful situation – parents with kids with special needs, people in stressful work situations, people in refuges, people with abusive partners... lots of people whose stress is unrelenting and who have no time for themselves. Stillness may not be an option for you right now, but my hope is that one day it will, or a few ideas might be inspiring to you even if you cannot put them into practice right now.

A good starting point if you are struggling (and know that we all do, at some point), is to nurture self-acceptance. Not judging or criticising yourself for doing the best you can in deeply challenging situations. Let's work towards a recognition that your feelings are true and valid. And not to feel guilty about how you are feeling, however you are feeling, viewing your experience instead as a point to start a journey of listening, accepting and learning.

Learning to rest on this journey, without feeling guilty, is a big step and can take time. But it can be done in little ways, wherever you are, whatever situation you are in: being out in nature, taking a short walk, closing your eyes and taking five deep breaths – these things are wonderful examples of what we call in Sanskrit *smarana*, remembering. Remembering to take time, remembering who we are, remembering the pace that works for us. Even in short moments.

In taking time to reconnect to ourselves, to the peace deep within us below the intense surface emotions and stresses, we also reconnect to inspiration, creativity and the courage to be our best selves under our own rules and values, not those portrayed to us.

The practices in this book will help you to remember another way of living. These can sustain us through the stressors that lie outside of our control. They can help us experience stillness on a regular basis, help us bring more calm to every situation we find ourselves in during our daily lives, and ask new questions of ourselves. Not 'how can I be bigger or faster?', not 'how much harder can I push?' but rather:

How can I live more simply?

How can I rest more deeply?

How easy can I make life for myself (and others)?

How can I embody calm?

Yin Magic

The concept of yin brings a framework and language that we seem to be lacking within our Western culture, which is why I'm reaching outside of it, for an established philosophical approach that can capture this vital part of life that we have omitted from our current way of being.

Yin is receptiveness, stillness, calm – and finding this element within our bodies and minds is absolutely magic… more than that, it is a superpower. When we are calm, our entire body functions more efficiently: we heal, digest, recover, think, breathe better. I call the relaxation response and yin, its 'own special magic'.

We will explore many practices here together through the lens of what I am calling yin magic: practices such as yin yoga, meditation, mindfulness and slow spells.

Imagine a great big beautiful tree: this is our yin magic tree! The roots are where we will start in this book. The first chapters explore the history of yin in the context of its native culture: Taoist alchemy, cosmology and Chinese medicine, so you can understand where many of these ideas that yin yoga was built on, are coming from. I think that's important. Now, these roots are huge and fascinating, and I will just offer a tiny glimpse from my understanding and encourage you to read more around the topics that interest you.

From these roots grows a sturdy trunk, as we draw energy and inspiration from the roots to look at how we can create a solid practice of yin yoga magic. We will explore its development and begin to practise yin yoga and yin energy magic in its many forms. Yin as a yoga practice is a practice of turning inwards. It is a practice of still, slow postures… often seemingly doing nothing. But there's strength here.

Once we get to the branches, we'll touch on magic, yoga, ritual and work with goddesses within and beyond their cultures of origin, as tools to use as we seek balance and yin in our own way. These magical and yogic practices can spread out into further branches and pathways and can be used on whatever path you are exploring.

I believe that 'slowness' is a power that we can and must bring to our magic because the modern need for speed has invaded this practice too. A while back, I picked up a book called *5-Minute Magic for Modern Wiccans: Rapid rituals, efficient enchantments, and swift spells*. I was struck by the word associations – to be modern is to be speedy, swift and efficient. I am very keen to represent a counter idea – of slow magic: easeful rituals, gentle enchantment and leisurely spells, as well as magic to be found within the process of slowing down and being still. Not as a 'better' option, but merely a different one, something that maybe we can embrace, so that we can have options to take things slowly when the mood takes us, or seek it out in our practice. This is the heart of yin magic.

My Journey to Yin

I love to tell stories, I love to listen to them too. I often tell my students the story, just as they settle down into *savasana* (relaxation), of the first time I went to a yoga class at age seven. When the time came for relaxation, I was wrapped in a blanket by the teacher's kindly helpers, tucked in on my mat. And I loved it. I tell my students that all I'm really trying to do in every class I teach is to recreate just a little of that feeling for my students: of being held, grounded, safe. So simple, but so powerful.

This is yin to me: the earth, the grounding, the roots, the connection, listening, knowing.

Since those first days of my early yoga practice, I've journeyed through Iyengar, hatha, vinyasa, kundalini, and yin yoga classes finding lessons and joy within them all. But when I wrote *Yoga for Witches* and tried to fit my love of yin into one chapter called Yin Magic... I knew this yin needed more! And it became a whole book! So this book is a love letter to yin, and to the joy of finding our own yin, and the beauty of finding gratitude and abundance in each moment.

Yin nourishes, it nurtures space for letting go. It asks: *What if we allowed ourselves to be guided by kindness, patience, and awareness?* In our practice and in life. Instead of by pressure to conform, compare, to meet standards and deadlines and invisible markers of success? *What if we simply sought peace and connection?* It's these ideas that draw a yoga class from simply movement of the body into the magical, the embodied spirituality of a yoga practice as spell, ritual, manifestation and intention.

My yoga and my yin yoga has allowed me to be... me. In the moment, nothing more, nothing less. And that's played a huge part in my own yin journey of acceptance of who I am, exactly as I am.

Old Traditions… New Practices

I love integrating practices and making connections between them.

My first book, *Yoga for Witches*, explored how to weave the Eastern wisdom of yoga philosophy into the practice of witchcraft, including my own Western magical practice, which is one of simple healing and connection to the rhythms of the natural world.

If this approach is new to you, I offer the following from *Yoga for Witches* by way of introduction:

Yoga is an embodied spiritual practice: moving the body, using intention and focused breathing to guide our movements. Yoga is a kind of ritual; each yoga asana (pose) not only moves the physical body but also opens the body's energy in its various forms. Witchcraft is, well, not so very different: a spiritual practice, that involves intention and focus. But also, a practice of creation and connection to spiritual and natural realms and cycles…

Uniting yoga with witchcraft allows us to create tangible experiences with the energy that connects our universe. Yoga for Witches is an exploration of how these two spiritual disciplines can be combined and explored to find greater peace, power and magic in our lives.

I'm bringing back that approach in this book too. We will be focusing on yin, both the concept in Chinese medicine and its history and philosophy within Taoism. We will explore how it has been honed for the West by yoga teachers in the last thirty years through the practice of yin yoga and how it might be consciously integrated with Western magical practices. In combining traditions and ideas, it is my intention to create something that may be greater than its individual parts: an embodied practice to help us live well in the midst of a busy culture.

This is the second book on the Yoga for Witches journey, as we continue to explore and combine various styles of yoga, witchcraft and cultural philosophies, all with the intention of guiding us to embody and embrace stillness. With some elements of yogic philosophy and witch lore – such as the Limbs of Yoga and the chakras – I'm going to assume some basic prior knowledge. If you'd like to go back and find those foundations or refresh your memory on Patanjali's *Yoga Sutras*, Ayurveda and kitchen witchcraft you can find out more in my previous book, *Yoga for Witches*.

Just as I love creating new ideas and weaving things together. I also love to reinforce that there is never just one way to approach a practice and embrace a philosophy – and that's true for yoga and for witchcraft. So, this is a presentation of some ideas that perhaps you've seen before, and some that you may find new: a selection of interesting ways to journey towards your yoga and magic work, your meditation and your stillness. This is your unique journey to wholeness, and I think that the more ideas you have, the more accurately you can plot your path on your journey.

I honour and deeply respect the wisdom that has gone before me. And I teach and write by drawing in my own experience and context and adding it to that which I have learned from the wisdom traditions of magic, yoga and Taoism. That's really the only way any of us can teach – to take what we've learned, wrap our own minds around it with our own thoughts and ideas, practice and embody it in our own lives, and then share our thoughts and reflections.

And yet, so often, with ideas of philosophy, religion, culture we can get caught up in rules and dogma and forget that all these systems were created by humans and continually changing with time and new ideas. Yoga, like many other ideas was created over thousands of years, with new influences constantly changing what 'yoga' was… incorporating ideas from Buddhist meditation, physical exercise and ritual practices. Along this timeline there is no one point where 'true' yoga emerged or existed. The same goes for a 'true' witchcraft or 'true' whatever. These traditions, ideas, and practices are fluid and ever-changing. It's a journey and a process. So, don't be scared to bring in your own ideas and influences.

In fact, I will be exploring several cultures that are not my own: Buddhist, Hindu and Chinese as well as my native cultures of Celtic, Saxon and Norse. As always, I strive to be humble and honest about my explorations, and never claim that I am something I'm not. I intend to share my knowledge and ideas, and always do so with utmost love and respect for the cultures and countries I am talking about.

Within the West, we are very often guilty of cultural appropriation or misappropriation: taking elements from a culture (such as the ideas of yin and yang) without taking the time to learn the deep meanings and significance of these elements. For example, you may see someone wearing a tee-shirt with the yin-yang symbol, *taijitu*, on it, that they bought in a fashionable store, but if you were to ask them they might not be able to tell you anything about the symbol, maybe they simply thought it a pretty image. (I'm not suggesting this person is in the wrong or had bad intentions, but the fashion industry is undoubtedly guilty of casual appropriation.)

There are topics within this book I know well, having studied and taught them for well over a decade: yoga, meditation and some sciences. There are some I have only started studying in earnest over the last few years: yin yoga and herb lore. And finally, there are some where I am little more than an enthusiastic amateur: such as Chinese medicine, Taoist philosophy and alchemy.

I am a passionate but imperfect guide, an ever-learning student, and encourage the same in you. Be curious, be humble, be respectful of traditions and creative in your approach. Research your sources and ideas, seek out those more knowledgeable than you. Live, love and learn wholeheartedly.

Beginner's Mind

Some people drawn to this book will be new to yoga, some to witchcraft, some to Taoism... and some to all of these ideas. My guess is that few will have explored the connections between the three at the same time.

If you are an expert in one of these fields, I invite you to come to this part of the practice, particularly, with what Zen Buddhists call "beginner's mind". Allow yourself to slow down, deepen into your practice and learn afresh... rather than to rush and skip forwards over these parts.

In my thirty years of yoga practice, I still struggle to let go of the pressure to, in some way, reflect my experience in poses. As such a long-time practitioner, should I not have mastered every asana? (I haven't. Not by a long way). When practicing as a child, it did not even occur to me that I should be seeking to 'master' a pose, and I try to carry that mentality with me. The practice is more than the pose.

Many of us have this idea that an advanced yogi is like something we have seen on Instagram: a muscly guy executing a one-handed Peacock Pose, or a flexible woman with both her legs behind her head. Some of these images *may* be of advanced practitioners. But it is more likely they are very skilled in the physical aspects of the yoga asana (some of the world's most famous Insta-yogis are former gymnasts and contortionists).

When I speak of yoga, that includes everything that yoga entails: not just physical asana, but also meditation, *pranayama*, self-care, service, self-study and right living. An advanced yogi is one who has mastered this eightfold path of Patanjali and released ego-bound desires and works consistently to still the fluctuations of body and mind.

Interestingly, most ancient images of advanced yogis and sages show them seated, often in *sukhasana* (Easy Seat) a pose that doesn't look that thrilling on Instagram! Easy Seat pose is one that I have genuine trouble getting my students to focus in, because many think it's simply a place to transition, to pause, barely a pose at all because it's so simple. For so long we have been conditioned that hard/impressive/elaborate = advanced, and easy/slow/soft = beginner. And so, I like to hold the image of the master yogis and gurus in my mind, proving, without meaning to, that Easy Seat is actually an advanced pose because the union of advanced yoga is happening within.

And I think witchcraft can hold some similarities – especially in traditional witching crafts of green witchery, spellcraft and kitchen witchery. Witches are practical people, they have to be. In the past they would have soothed wounds, aided childbirth, advised people and foretold events – things that needed doing. And yes, the ceremony would have been a part of that. Still, the practical witch had no time for showy extras: she used earth, herbs, stones because they were what was available to her. And she certainly wouldn't have been able to waste money on, for example, a fancy cloak or a bejewelled cauldron that made her look more 'advanced'. In fact, the reverse would be true: the more advanced the witch, the more quickly and easily she could call in her energy and set her focus, often without the need for props and tools at all.

The more advanced the practitioner, in my eyes, the more easeful and simple their practice becomes – what an advanced practitioner *really* doesn't give a fig about is what they look like.

Now, this is not a criticism to many of us who are enjoying working towards handstands and Scorpion Pose in yoga. And who have gathered an elaborate altar as, like magpies, we have collected many shiny delights and beautiful oracle decks and decadent incense (which I love!). It's a beautiful thing that the secrets of super-challenging poses are shared and supported. And that we live in a world (for the most part) that allows us to fly our witchy flag. And that we enjoy enough wealth to enjoy buying things that delight and inspire us, rather than just the bare essentials. But this is, I suppose, a reminder and something to think on.

It's always useful to consider pride and ego and remember why you are on this path of the witch, yogi or any other. In yoga, we can all, sometimes, lose sight of the real reason we came to the mat, and our practice is no longer about connecting to our bodies in the present moment but pushing ourselves into impressive asana. Or the mind is distracted with thoughts about how we could be better or stronger or in comparing ourselves to others. Patanjali warns that unity should be the sole goal of the yoga path, not the possession of power or praise.

Try and leave your ego out of the journey as best as you can. As the classic yoga text *Hatha Yoga Pradipika* tells us, it's the doing that matters "neither by wearing the garb of a Siddha nor by talking about it is perfection attained. Only through the practical application does one become a Siddha". To possess the power of the siddhis (yogic magical powers…one who has attained them is called a Siddha) don't show off, don't talk others down, don't seek followers to tell you how great you are – just do the work. If you are truly seeking enlightenment, your joys should and will lay within that. The joy of the practice itself is the greatest reward.

CLOSING YINSIGHTS

I am writing this book at a time that will be ingrained in our history. During the last few months, something big happened to force many of us to slow down in some way: the coronavirus lockdown of 2020. Lots of us not on the front line or with intense caring roles experienced a different mode of being, an enforced slowing down. A new pace of life and different challenges were presented to us.

Whilst the virus has had a horrific impact on individuals, families and communities, lockdown itself could be considered a gift in some ways – inviting us to pause and reflect. My grandmother, who up to this point was still working long hours, has found more time to spend in her garden. My mother has taken to walking by the sea. Simple practices they sometimes previously felt too busy to do, or simply forgot was an option.

On the other hand, however, spending lots of time at home is not necessarily a lovely relaxing holiday. We are stressed, we are worried, and we are fearful. When we remove the busyness of our commutes, shopping, social events – we are left with a new practice: grappling with our own minds. What happens without constant life distractions? What can come from stillness? From silence? If we are able to ask these questions now or at any time, and confront the feelings that arise, we are given an opportunity to know what it means to be present.

To live with yin is to live mindfully and with intention.

I believe that living with yin presents a solution to the sense of rush, busyness, overwhelm and inability to slow down that many of us experience. I invite you to explore this yin magic with me within these pages. And I also invite you to take your time on the journey! It is always useful to remind ourselves that we are all walking our own path at our own pace, and that complicated, and challenging does not equate to advanced practice or guarantee enlightenment.

So, take your time: this is your journey – no need to put pressure on yourself here!

I invite you to put down the book before starting the next chapter and allow yourself to get back into your body and the world beyond it. The following are a few very simple ideas to start you off with little or no equipment, training or fancy clothing and no philosophy to understand. Why not try one of these, now, without expectation?

Choose one that is suitable for wherever you are right now. You might want to set a 10-minute timer on your phone so that you are not worrying about time (or rushing!).

- Journal or free write – about your day, your year, or anything that comes to mind.
- Light a candle and watch it burn – see if you can bring your attention to its form, shape and movement.
- Gaze out of the window – note movements and colours.
- Meditate – use your breath as a point of focus.
- Massage your hands and feet using a scented oil or lotion.
- Stand in nature (whether in your garden, on the beach, in a forest or wherever you can find).

2

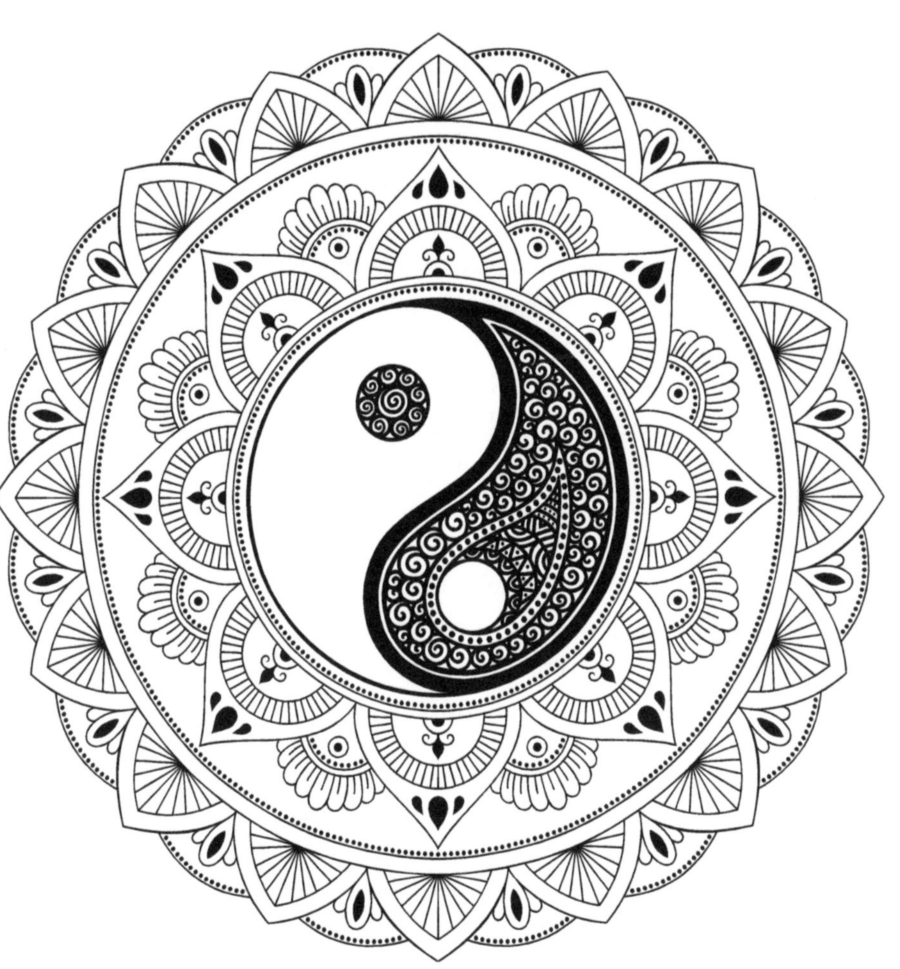

THE STORY OF YIN

In the beginning there was... yin (and yang!). In the Chinese story of creation, it all began with yin and yang. From their home at the centre of the earth as polarised energies they gave birth to the universe and its energy: *qi*. From here came the first humans and deities. This polarity of yin and yang – and their connection to absolutely everything – is at the very roots of Chinese philosophy and culture.

These ideas of yin and yang were put to paper in such beautiful ancient texts as the world's oldest medical book, *Huangdi Neijing*, the Yellow Emperor's Book of Medicine, during the third millennium BCE; the *I Ching* (*The Book of Changes*, a text of divination) around 800 BCE; and the *Tao Te Ching* (around 400 BCE). All three of these great texts in some way present yin, yang and *qi* as an understanding of the movement and expression of energy throughout humans, nature and universe, and the continuous process of change, within which balance can be found.

The ideas encapsulated in these texts are that the universe is composed of forces of yin and yang, *qi* and the five *wu xing* elements (I'll talk more about these shortly). These elements affect the macrocosm of the world, and equally the microcosm of the human. And in understanding these natural forces, a person can find balance and health: illness being caused by imbalance of these forces in some way. Chinese medicine seeks to help create this inner state and life of balance, harmonising the body, mind, emotions, and spirit, and an individual's energy with nature. Just as witches say: "as above, so below".

All things carry yin and embrace yang.
They reach harmony by blending with the vital breath.
The Tao Te Ching, Lao Tzu

Everything contains yin and yang. They are two opposite, yet complimentary, energies. Yin is a receptive energy that compliments yang's creative energy, making a complete whole. All natural dualities – sun and moon, day and night, light and dark, expansion and contraction – are physical manifestations of the interconnectedness of yin and yang. The principle of yin and yang is represented by the *taijitu*, what we call in the West; the yin yang symbol. Within this symbol we see something elemental, all at once incredibly simple and incredibly complex.

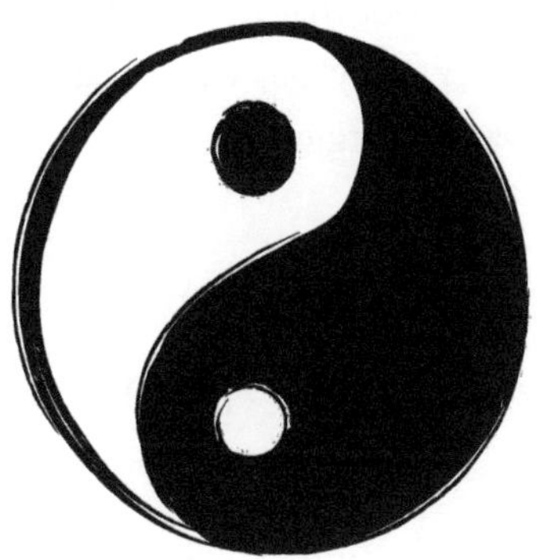

The dots within each of the two sides represent that there is always some yin (black) within yang (white) and vice versa. Each half of the circle will always contain some yin and some yang. There are no absolutes. Taking the example of night and day, we can see that night is yin and day is yang. However, within every day there is both a yang part (the rising and midday sun) and a yin part (dusk, as day turns to night).

Pairs of these two universal energies

Yang	—	Yin	Energy	—	Matter
Heaven	—	Earth	Activity	—	Rest
Sun	—	Moon	Rising	—	Descending
Firm	—	Yielding	East	—	West
Light	—	Darkness	South	—	North
Fire	—	Water	Male	—	Female
Time	—	Space			

Remember, in our focus here on yin, that it's not about one or other. It's not about getting rid of yang, but finding the balance between them. As we live in a very yang culture, I'm working on the hypothesis that many of us could do with some additional yin in our lives to find our balance. We seek the inner *'yuj'* – yoking of our yin and yang sides – *yuj* is the Sanskrit root that the word yoga originates from. So just as we seek to connect in yoga, we can also seek to connect and balance our yin and yang energies.

YIN AND TAOISM

Man follows Earth
Earth follows Heaven
Heaven follows the Tao
And the Tao follows Nature[i]

***The Tao Te Ching*, Lao Tzu**

When Lao Tzu explored yin and yang in his book; the *Tao Te Ching*, he also presented a philosophy, that he called the Tao – 'The Way'. The *Tao Te Ching* became one of the foundational texts of the Taoist path – sharing that the key to a long healthy life is to follow the Tao, which is the natural flow of the universe. Like Patanjali's yoga sutras, the idea of Tao existed before Lao Tzu, but he created a guide that is one of the most well-known, especially to us here in the West.

Lao Tzu describes Tao as like water: flowing, soft yet powerful, nourishing all things.[ii] To live with Tao is to find harmony in the natural rhythm of life. Though the universe is in a state of constant

---

i So closely linked are Tao and nature that in some translations of the *Tao Te Ching*, that last line is written, as 'Tao follows itself'.

ii You will see a lot of water imagery connected to Tao and the meridians. Water is a yin element.

flux. That in-between place, the flowing centre of finding balance of yin, yang, *qi* and *wu xing*, that point of equilibrium, that harmony, that's the Way, that's the Tao.

In Tao (and this will look very familiar to both yoga and witchcraft practitioners) everything is connected, nothing and no one are separate. Using yin and yang again as an example, light and dark are connected and inseparable, moving in a cycle. We cannot have the light without the dark, we cannot have day without night. Furthermore, neither of these sides are good or bad, because they are inseparable parts of one whole.

Tao, like yoga, is a journey toward peace. Effortlessness and simplicity lie at the heart of its practices. In accordance with Tao, one has to 'do nothing' (known as *wu wei* – effortless action). Nothing, that is, against the tide of nature. In yoga, we embrace a very similar idea called 'effortless effort' finding a peacefulness even in challenging poses, because we are always moving with mindfulness and in harmony with our own body and breath.

Over time, Taoist ideas have mixed with Confucianism, folk tradition and Buddhism, making a beautiful, magical blend that varies through Chinese culture. I think all these threads woven together make for a rich mix, and a nourishing and varied practice. Some who follow Tao as a concept focus more on the internal work of following the Way, some seek to connect to ancestors and ritual. As always, there's no right or wrong, simply the way you find it, and a call to explore as we find our own Way.

Basic Tao Concepts of Internal Energy

All things hold energy in the Taoist universe, and a concept central to Taoism and Chinese medicine is that harmony can be reached by working with the three forms of energy in the body. *Shen*, *jing* and *qi*; known as the *san bao* – three treasures – are the foundations of sustaining life, each one contributing to overall health and wellbeing of the body.

Shen

Shen or 'spirit' is our higher self: the part of us that is divine and connected to the energy of the universe. Usually visualised around the head, *shen* is our mind, responsible for our consciousness, wisdom, awareness and emotions. Influencing activities that take place in the mental, spiritual, and creative realms. Through our shen, we radiate our energy into the world. *Shen* can be harmed by unhealthy habits (all the usual culprits: chips, booze, smoking…) as well as through internal elements, such as self-criticism. Disharmony of *shen* may manifest itself as anxiety, insomnia or depression.

Jing

Our 'essence', *jing* is seed energy that forms the root of who we are. It is thought to reside in the kidneys and/or pelvic area. Our primal life force, *jing* is a foundational and finite energy resource, and it is this energy that determines one's lifespan (although one can cultivate *jing* from healthy living, it's a little different, known as 'acquired *jing*'). *Jing* is passed down to us from and through our ancestors, so this seed may also hold memory or attributes passed down through generations. *Jing* depletion can result in such issues as adrenal exhaustion and infertility.

Qi

Qi (pronounced *chee*, and also spelt 'chi') is the life force or the 'breath of life' that animates and controls the functions of all living beings. It is located in and around the chest: lungs, diaphragm and heart. Being close to the heart, it is also connected to emotions. *Qi* in humans is drawn from the air we breathe and the food we eat, action and intention also play a role. *Qi* flows through the body in energy channels known as meridians that connect all of our major organs. Disease can arise when the flow of *qi* in the meridians becomes unbalanced or blocked. Any pain or illness can represent an obstruction in the normal flow of *qi* through the energy lines of the body.

Qi's counterpart in other cultures (not direct translations but similar ideas of life force) include:

Hindu philosophy: *prana*
Polynesian: *mana*
Egyptian: *ka*
Greek: *pneuma*
Druidry: *awen*

WU XING – THE FIVE ELEMENTS

In its perpetual journey, *qi* travels through five elements or phases *(wu xing)* – Fire, Water, Metal, Wood and Earth. *Wu xing* (pronounced *woo zing*) means: 'five types of *qi* that govern at different times', but that's a little long, so we tend to shorten it to just 'five elements'! What we are looking at is a conceptual framework of natural dynamism that can describe anything from season to organs to personality types and relationships.

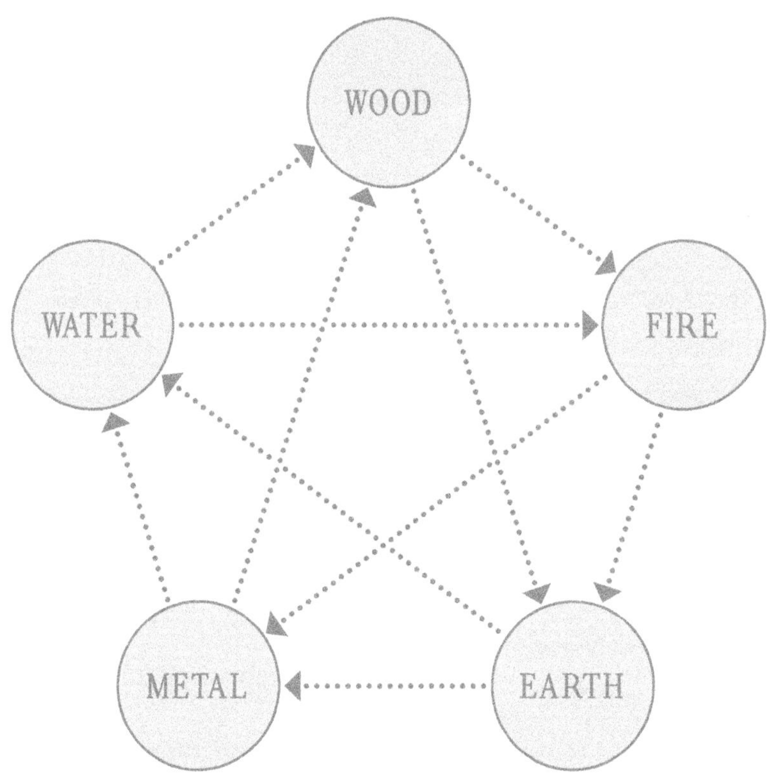

Although we often call *wu xing* the 'five elements' in English, *wu xing* are very different to our Western understanding of the elements of earth, air, fire and water. *wu xing* transcend the literal/tangible objects of earth or water. Really the *wu xing* have more in common with the Ayurvedic[iii] ideas of elements and doshas referred to in yogic practice, which represent change and purpose.

The *wu xing* elements interact with each other in countless ways: nurturing, destroying and weakening. For example, Water destroys Fire but allows Wood to grow, Metal is born from Earth and both Earth and Metal can hold Water. This diagram illustrates the two major cycles of the generative and the destructive phases.

The generative (sometimes known as mother) phases go around the outside.

- Wood feeds Fire
- Fire creates Earth
- Earth produces Metal
- Metal holds Water
- Water nourishes Wood

The overcoming or destructive (often known as father) phases go across the circle.

- Wood parts Earth (think roots)
- Earth dams (or muddies) Water
- Water extinguishes Fire
- Fire melts Metal
- Metal cuts Wood

iii Ayurveda is an ancient Indian healing modality very closely connected with yoga. For more on it see *Yoga for Witches*.

Pentagram

You'll see how the lines that connect the elements create a pentagram. This five-pointed star has been used symbolically since Ancient Babylonia and Mesopotamia, and is found in Pagan and earth-based religions, including witchcraft. It can be used to represent, amongst other things: the five senses, five elements and five points of the human body – feet, hands and head.

Seasons, people, emotions, positive and negative behaviour, moods and ailments can all be addressed relative to the five elements. We contain all *wu xing* elements, but variables such as inherent nature, environment and situations can influence which are dominant. One or two elements may be dominant in a person (just as with the Ayurvedic doshas). They can influence our individual physical, mental, and emotional character traits as well as our unique powers and weaknesses. Simple awareness of our leading *wu xing* energy can help guide our practice and bring knowledge to where we may struggle or meet imbalance.

CORRESPONDENCES

Each of the *wu xing* elements correlates to specific organs in the body, a season, colour and either yin or yang dominance. These can be laid out in tables of correspondence (connected concepts that cluster together) which we often use in Western witchcraft.

In the vein of sympathetic magic, 'like affects like'. So if we feel lacking in energy and want to connect to the rising energy of Fire, we may use the colour red and connection to the heart in a spell – as they are connected to energy of Fire in Chinese wisdom. Whereas if someone has too much Fire energy dominant within them, they may feel anger, overwhelm or an inability to settle. A Chinese medicine or acupuncture practitioner may address an imbalance by overcoming Fire with Water: unblocking or encouraging the Water meridian, or prescribing drinking more water, as well as avoiding very hot weather (or very hot yoga studios!) that would stoke Fire further. A witch or yogi may connect to watery elements for a similar effect with correspondence such as blue crystals or deities of water.

Wu Xing Correspondences

Wood *(mu)*

Season: Spring. The *qi* energy of the Wood element is most prominent in the spring when plants are sprouting new growth during this season of energy and vitality.

Yin/yang: Yang. **Colour:** Green.

Meridian Channels and Organs: Liver and Gallbladder.

Animal Correspondence: Rabbit and dragon – grounded but springy! Both can take flight in their own way. Rabbits are a symbol of hope and long life in Taoism. I'm particularly fond of the Chinese folk tale which says that the grey shapes we can see on the moon are the form of the rabbit familiar of Moon Goddess, Chang'e. The moon rabbit keeps her company while she mixes the elixir of immortality from her lunar home.

Personality Type: Wood personalities are full of ideas and enthusiasm. They love to push limits and boundaries, to stretch and reach tall. Wood personality may see a yogi that holds a pose that looks beautiful, but they may have trouble quietening their thoughts, that can branch out in all directions. If you find this, you could visualise your thoughts drawing back down to earth, and to your roots. Or as Metal can overcome wood (like an axe carving a tree trunk), work on focusing on your breath, lungs being connected to the Metal element.

Fire *(huo)*

Season: Summer. The season of the Fire element; rising, swelling energy when the weather is hottest. A time of healing, health and joy.

Yin/yang: Yang. **Colour:** Red.

Meridian Channels and Organs:
Heart and Small Intestines. Pericardium and Triple Burner.

Animal Correspondence: Red birds and the phoenix, as well as beetles, which represent rebirth and transformation.

Personality Type: Fire people are energetic, warm, creative, and passionate. A Fire personality yogi is vibrant and loves to chat with their friends in a yoga class but they can have trouble settling into long held, cool, yin poses. Water puts out flames, so, a focus on Kidney and Bladder meridians can help (I'll go through yoga poses that can do this in the next chapter). Earth smothers Fire, so grounding poses like Child's Pose can be useful to help ease your Fire to warm embers instead of wild flames.

Earth *(tu)*

Season: Each *wu xing* element is dominant in a particular season, and while the Earth element is connected to late summer, it also features in every season as an ever-present grounding energy. In some schools of thought as the transitory phase between each season, energy and movement come back "Home" to earth before it moves out again into the next phase. Mother Earth is a central point around which the seasons and the elements turn.

Yin/yang: Yin. **Colour:** Yellow.

Meridian Channels and Organs: Stomach and Spleen.

Animal Correspondence: Cow – abundant and nurturing.

Personality Type: Earth personalities are nurturing, compassionate and peaceful, but can become caught within furrows of worry and anxiety. Wood can overcome Earth, parting it with solid roots and rising from it. This can be done through a connection to Liver and Gallbladder in a forward fold for example. Or channel hopeful Wood energy by setting new intentions *(sankalpa)* for your practice.

Metal *(jin)*

Season: Autumn. The time of harvesting the abundance of summer, and a transition time from the heat and light of summer into colder seasons. The energy here is of letting go, like leaves falling off a tree as it draws energy reserves inwards to its trunk. This is a time for letting go of what is no longer vital, slowing down, gathering and storing what is needed for winter.

Yin/yang: Yin. **Colour:** White.

Meridian Channels and Organs: Lungs and Large Intestine.

Animal Correspondence: Horse and Tiger: strong, steadfast, solid and holding, horses and tigers are yin.

Personality Type: Metal energy people like definition and structure. As a personality; Metal, whilst it can be used to 'cut away' what no longer serves us, may in imbalance, try to keep emotions and feelings contained. The great inner strength of Metal personality can find it hard to let go. Fire melts Metal, so creating warmth, with a heart focused practices can support release. Outside of the studio just bringing yourself to a warm space like a soothing bath can help. (Water can rust Metal so it too may help break down some boundaries).

Water *(shui)*
Season: Winter. Winter is connected to the Water element, and the cold creates a time for hibernation: plants go into their dormant cycle, and animals and humans retreat into their homes, storing their energy for the spring to come. The yin Water element of this season invites us to engage in nourishing activities and connect to the flow of life.

Yin/yang: Yin. **Colour:** Black/dark blue.

Meridian Channels and Organs: Kidneys and Bladder.

Animal Correspondence: Fish – serenity and bravery.

Personality Type: Water people are introspective, seekers of knowledge and understanding. But this introspection can lead to fear and anxiety. Earth can overcome Water, holding it as a dam, so grounding yoga poses, grounding spell work, and/or connection to the Stomach and Spleen meridian can help reduce fear in someone with too much Water energy.

SEASONAL LIVING

Our lives can be thrown off balance by a lack of stillness, but also in trying to fight with the energy inherent in the seasons. Sometimes we are so used to organising our lives with our 9 to 5, 5 days a week, 365 days a year lifestyles, that we can forget that there are seasons that bring out different feelings and phases within us. Do we dedicate so much time to sprouting and blooming with Wood and Fire that we don't have time to ground and rejuvenate with yin energy of Earth and Water? Or are we stuck in the hibernation of winter, Water and worry, unable to find our fiery spark?

We can observe the five elements and their correspondences in our own lives. If you are finding your habits or even your favourite pastimes unenjoyable, challenging or draining, it might help to explore if they are aligned or in conflict with the elemental energy of the season and of your own nature. Drawing on these ideas of phases of elemental energy gives us a chance to explore what elements are prevalent in our own lives and which may need nurturing or overcoming. For example, it may be a cultural standard in the West to set New Year's resolutions in January, but your energy is still in winter yin, many of us would have more success taking on new habits by waiting to sprout and grow with the Wood in spring! Or if you are a Fire personality, taking hot yoga classes in high summer may be a fiery overload that overwhelms and leaves you stressed. This is an invitation to look at how you can tailor your routines to fit the season.

Sometimes we try and force habits, and that can cause stress. The same goes for socialising – if you are an Earth personality you may find walking through town into busy pubs joyful in summer as people spill out on the street, energised by the longer nights. But in winter, you may find the flow of good conversation with friends at home more soothing and nourishing to your *qi*.

So, to end this chapter, we will explore a simple yin practice of connecting with elemental energy to help us find some stillness.

5 Element Meditation

Take the five-element meditation posture by lying on the ground – spread your legs and arms out like a starfish, creating the five points of the pentagram symbol with your body.

- Take some deep easeful breaths and gently close the eyes.
- Take another deep breath in, breathing deep into the belly. As you breathe out become aware of your body and bones settling. The Earth element of the body connecting to the Earth that supports us here. Grounded and rooted like a mountain, able to withstand all the challenges life brings your way. Drawing

groundedness and stability into your stomach as it rises and falls with deep easeful breaths. Perhaps envisage yourself resting in a forest clearing, or meadow with a view of a beautiful mountain, with golden yellow sunlight shining upon you.

- Allow your lungs to take in air. The Metal element is the element of the lungs, imagine a shiny or silvery light. The lungs are like silver chalices holding this precious breath. And swirling sparkling light that you draw in, moves around your chest and head.
- The breath moves like the rhythm of water, like the lapping of a blue lake along a shoreline or the gentle trickle of a woodland stream as we connect to the Water element. Perhaps we envisage the water washing over our legs and belly, maybe we dangle our feet in it or take a paddle.
- Above you, trees wave and sway, soft and green, leaves dancing in the breeze. With the element of Wood, you feel connected to the energy blooming within you like saplings, rising and growing at their own pace. You feel a peaceful power in this place of nature, unhurried, yet vibrantly alive.
- Draw all this energy and light inwards towards the heart space now, the Fire element. Imagine it filling up your heart with warm red light, and overflowing to fill your whole body with light and easeful power.
- Feel the five elements blend within you and blending with the perfect balance of the Tao/spirit/universe.

CLOSING YINSIGHTS

The elements and energy outlined in Chinese culture represent journeys of constant flux and transformation. We do not always welcome change, but something new and beautiful is happening with every step on our journey. The truth that nothing is constant, is woven deeply into Chinese philosophy. Within the ideas of *wu xing*, yin and yang are an opportunity to change, regroup, refresh, settle and balance – a framework that we can utilise to support the rhythm of our lives.

None of us are just one thing, we change moment to moment – it is no wonder that stillness and slowness can be a challenge. What we need and what our rest looks like can change from day to day. That uncertainty can be a little daunting, but it is a gift! Every day, every moment, is an opportunity to reconnect with your stillness, to find your way back to centre, which, according to Lao Tzu is essential to finding your path and your 'Way'.

3

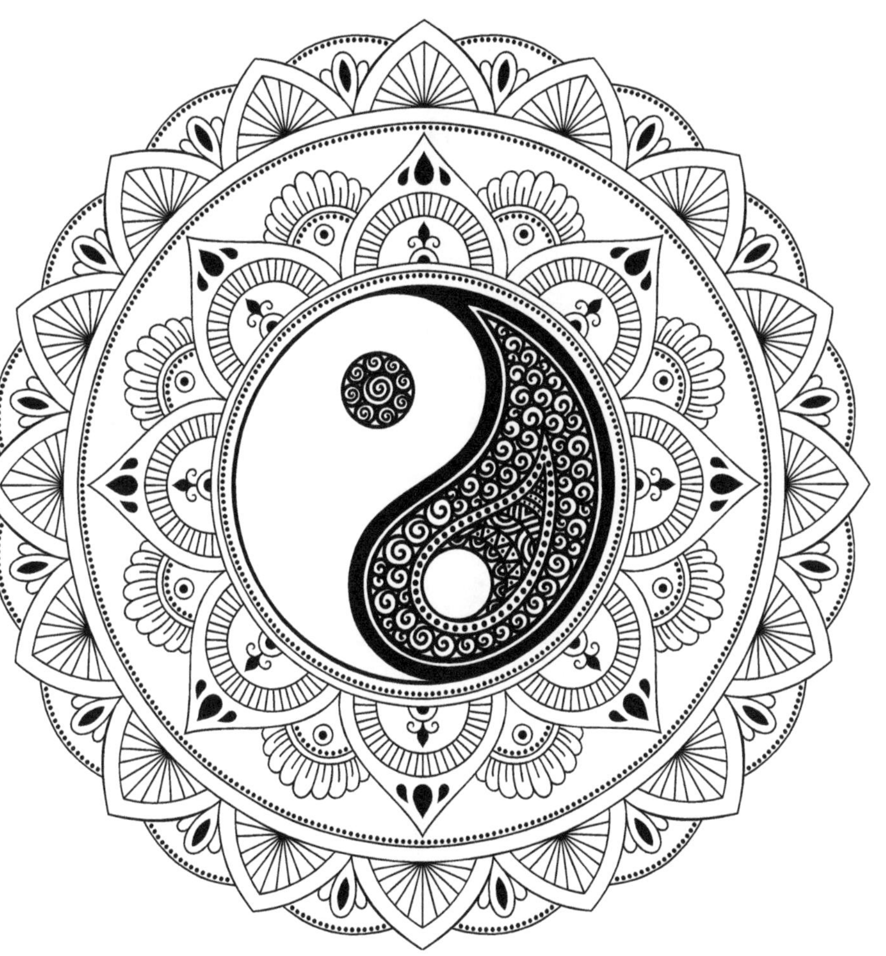

YIN YOGA

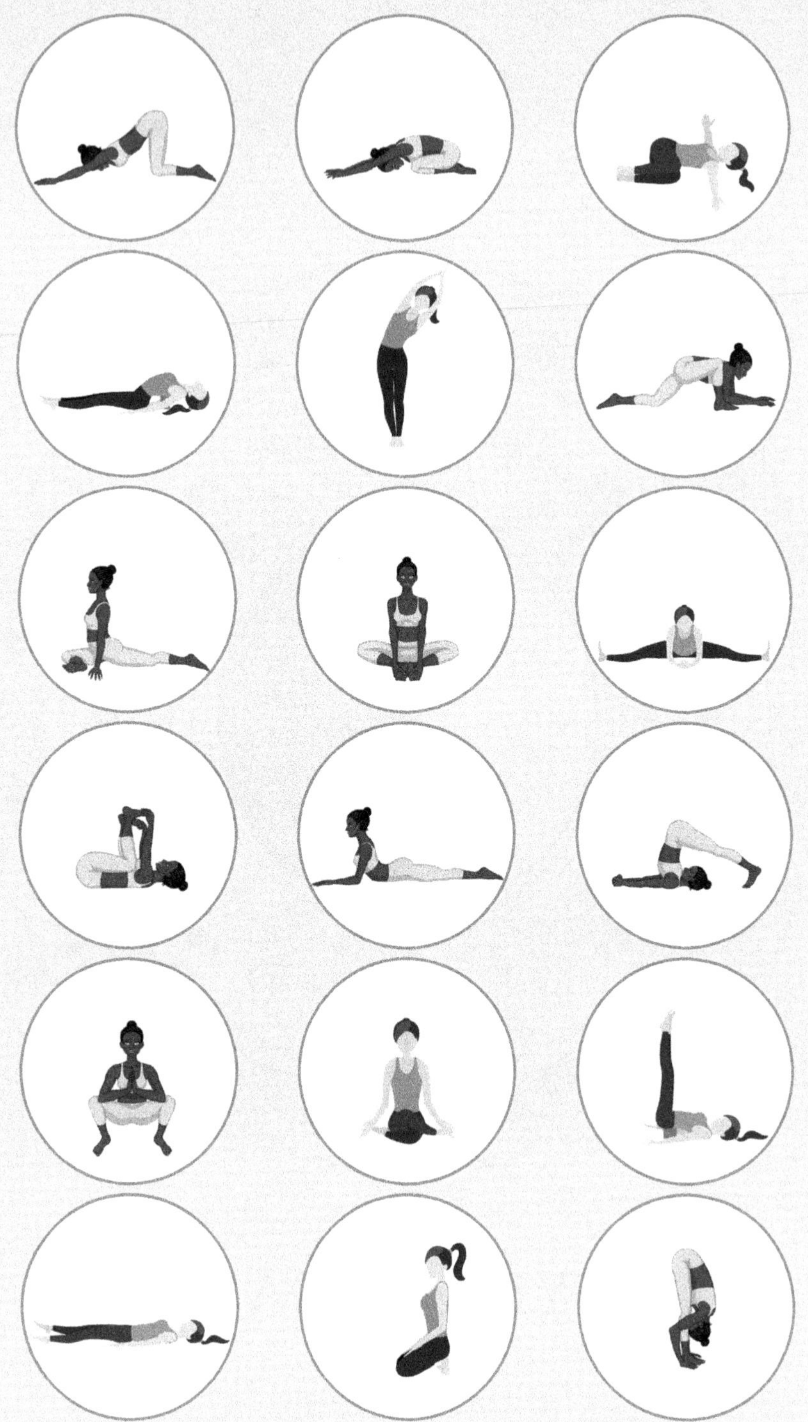

The benefits from yin yoga are not purely physical: students also benefit from the stillness the practice offers.
Bernie Clarke, *The Complete Guide to Yin Yoga*

We've journeyed through yin and yang, through earth, water, fire, wood and metal, just some of the key ideas from Taoism, Chinese medicine and alchemy from which the practice of yin yoga was drawn.

The actual term "yin yoga" was coined around 1990: it's a modern invention built from ancient practices. And one of the many joys of yin yoga being a recent creation is that the teachers who developed this style of practice – Paulie Zink, Paul Grilley, Sarah Powers, Bernie Clarke and Norman Blair – are available to study and practice with right now.

Yin yoga is best known for its slowness and long-held stretches, though these are not unique to yin yoga of course, and are found in many other physical disciplines, from martial arts to gymnastics and ballet, mainly for increasing flexibility. In hatha yoga, B. K. S. Iyengar (celebrated twentieth century yoga teacher and guru) recommended holding *supta virasana* (Reclining Hero Pose) for 10–15 minutes (my knees couldn't handle that!). Yoga has, from its Hindu roots, always been a practice for moving into stillness. And yin yoga; invites us to move even deeper into this stillness.

There are only around twenty yin yoga poses (specific poses and styles vary from teacher to teacher), which is more than enough as you'll likely do no more than a handful in each yin yoga class. This can be a change to those used to rattling through lots and lots of different asana during yoga practice. You will notice that yin yoga poses have different names to those you may be familiar with from hatha or vinyasa yoga practice. Because yin yoga was created by native English speakers, the names of yin yoga poses are in English, and very little Sanskrit is used.[i] We are approaching these poses in our yin style,

i If your teacher is, like me, trained in classical hatha yoga – the odd Sanskrit/hatha word may sneak in!

and so this shift in language helps us to view the poses and practice in a different way. For example, in classical hatha yoga pose *baddha Konasana,* which translates from Sanskrit as 'bound angle pose' – is called Butterfly in yin; so, it's not just that it's an English translation of the pose's name, but we are approaching the pose from a whole different viewpoint. Like all good magic, it's about intention. And you won't find strong standing poses like *Virabhadrasana* (Warrior Pose) – because they are too yang for this style of practice.

The combination of ancient Indian traditions with Chinese theories of energy meridians in the body enhance the benefits of yoga as well as provide deeper insights into how the body works. This helps to harmonise the body, balancing the emotions, bringing us into a connection with the true nature of our being and the rhythm and flow of nature (Tao). In yin yoga, specific yoga postures are used to channel the energetic attributes of yin and yang, and to stimulate the transformational properties of the five alchemical elements.

Yin yoga exerts a slow, steady force on the body – namely gravity. The long-held poses (3-5 minutes) of yin yoga do not require much muscular strength. The magic happens on deeper, subtler levels of the connective tissues: fascia, ligaments and joints, by holding a yin pose we find space in muscles and stimulate connective tissue. In finding this space we are getting into some of those dark corners of the body. (In Chapter 8 I'll talk about the magical dark as a place for healing and transformation).

Cool Yoga – a Contrast to Hot Yoga

Yang is heat and fire. Its movement creates heat in the body – aerobics, running and some high energy forms of yoga, such as vinyasa yoga are very yang. In our culture we are encouraged to build a sweat and feel the burn. Hot yoga classes, popularised in fast-paced cities around the US and Europe, are the ultimate yang – high temperatures, intense asanas and sometimes something of a gruelling ethos.

Yin is about finding stillness, soothing and cooling the body. We aren't generating heat in the body in our yin yoga postures. Instead, we settle into the cool and the dark. We embody the feminine moon energy of slow yin, rather than the fiery masculine energy of yang.

Yin yoga practice allows time within each pose to observe bodily sensations and mental processes. It works with the yoga practice of using postures to help the body and mind sit more easefully in meditation, which is generally considered to be a yin activity.

Yin yoga is hugely beneficial to those who have been stoking the flames of yang in their lives for so long. If we focus only on the yang, the body can suffer from fatigue and burnout. Too much heat and we burn. We might feel the sparks of pain in the body or the 'hot-headedness' of anger, frustration and stress.

Yin invites us to cool the flames in stillness. Here we can rest, recharge, relax, soothing stress, anxiety and overwhelm, as well as stretching tense muscles and overworked bodies. When we do so, we release the emotional stresses that are held, according to Chinese medicine, within the tissues of the body.

Getting Into your Comfort Zone

The comfort zone has got some bad press of late, with calls for people to push out of their comfort zone in the name of self-improvement. Even yin yoga teachers can nurture this idea of the value of settling with discomfort, physically and/or emotionally. And don't get me wrong taking on challenges is great, and yes, working with our edges and facing fears is a way to grow. But there is much to be said for the comfort zone. And of course, a balance.

Moments of challenge through the day can be exciting, but if you find yourself in a constant state of fear, anxiety or overwhelm, then I believe seeking your comfort zone may be just the ticket. As my dear friend Eleni, a gifted counsellor, would say 'a nice dose of ordinary' can really help us heal, and rest. Finding joy in simple tasks, relaxing rituals and routines all invite this slowing down. And if you can find it during your yoga practice, you'll allow the body to relax, finding an edge of a nice stretch, but never reaching a place of pain or fear.

My Journey to Yin

It feels that much of my life has been yang. I've always found *savasana* (Pose of Relaxation) the toughest asana for me. Curiosity led me to a trusted teacher's yin class. I just about managed to get through the ninety minutes, but wriggled constantly and used immense will power to survive. However, I went back again and again as I sensed I needed this stillness in my body and in my life.

My week's immersive training with Norman Blair took it to a whole new level. His calmness was infectious, and his whole sense of being was settled. He was a human being, and I was a human doing! Since then, I have embraced curiosity and delved deeper into my own yin practice and developed my own way of sharing it with others and inviting my students to accept where they are physically, mentally, energetically and welcome all sensations around their being.

Trish, yin yoga teacher

Of course, as I said in the introduction many of us may feel 'scared to be still' and it may be more of a challenge to find our comfort zone within stillness. But this is just a reminder that faster, scarier, bigger, is not always better, instead it can lead us to greater damage to ourselves.

I invite you to take time in your comfort zone, with things that bring you calm. Unhurried cooking, reading a book, meditation, swimming in warm waters, picnicking, listening to birdsong, watching a cat sleep in the sun, gathering blackberries from hedgerows, sipping on fresh mint tea, and of course – easeful yin yoga! Allow your comfort zone to be a place you savour.

Learning to Let Go

All forms of yoga are not just what we do – the poses – but how we do them: the flow of energy and the mental attitude. Yin yoga is no different. In it, we learn to embody the practice of *wu wei*, the Taoist concept of 'non-action': the wisdom of when to hold on and when to let go. This always reminds me of my favourite Terry Pratchett quote, which I often share in the classes I teach:

> *There are times in life when people must know when not to let go. Balloons are designed to teach small children this.*

Yin yoga is a time to let go of the balloon! Through yin yoga, we can discover a feeling of peace through letting go, and from that place, compassion and loving-kindness towards ourselves can arise. Also, in learning when to let go, we can learn when to hold on as well, reserving our strength for when holding is needed.

WU WEI

When your body is not aligned,
The inner power will not come.
When you are not tranquil within,
Your mind will not be well ordered.
Align your body, assist the inner power,
Then it will gradually come on its own.

The Neiye [ii]

ii The *Neiye* (meaning Inward Training), are ancient Chinese texts describing Taoist breath meditation and *qi* circulation, from about 350 BCE.

Many artists, musicians, and writers know the state called 'flow' where everything simply comes together with ease – losing all sense of time we can tap into a channel of inspiration. Yoga practice also presents the opportunity to connect to flow. We can uncover moments in our yoga when we open ourselves to being completely present and deeply mindful.

The idea is that we can, and should, stop trying to force action, lies at the heart of what it means to follow Tao. In the *Tao Te Ching* this idea of *wu wei*, is explored as the 'action of non-action' or 'effortless action'. Some of the meaning of *wu wei* is illustrated when we talk of being 'in flow'. It's a surrender to the natural cycles of the world, but also carrying peace whilst being engaged in challenging tasks, so that one can carry these out with the most efficiency.

Wu wei, combined with yin is, I think, one of the essential concepts that can help us in finding stillness and harmony. It is a practice of profound acceptance: acceptance both of yourself, and your unfolding life.

Wu wei relates to our yoga as we work towards allowing our practice to unfold: inviting our body to move and open, rather than striving. It can be very tempting to force our practice as we try to grab and pull ourselves into a position, perhaps a little closer to the floor, or to our own toes... But in doing so, we are missing the point of the practice, one which is loving and compassionate, not competitive. This is known as equanimity, that state where no matter what's happening, we can view it from a place of calm. In cultivating *wu wei* and equanimity, we allow our practice to come to us, rather than setting a plan for where we want it to go. We learn to listen deeply and let go of how we think a pose is supposed to look, focusing instead on how our body can settle into a comfortable space within a pose with patience.

My Journey to Yin

The reason I love the practice of yin is that it opens your awareness to the subtleties that are often overlooked in a more yang style of practice. Staying in the poses for longer gives you a real sense of what is going on inside, not just physically but also psychologically and emotionally.

My favourite sensations to focus on in a yin practice are:

- the subtle waves of the breath that, combined with gravity, offer a gentle lifting and lowering quality to the inner body
- watching a particular sensation as it grows, shrinks, moves or spreads out around the body
- the way I react to being in a pose – this will depend entirely on my state of mind that day.

I credit this practice, and this practice alone, with teaching me patience. I used to be very impatient and would get bored and give up on things very quickly. I am far less reactionary than I ever was.

Yin invites us to stay with discomfort and observe what happens without reacting or moving straight away. I have found that I have transferred this into my life off the mat. The way that we are invited to stay, observe and soften the body, reactions and feelings in a pose or a situation has enabled me to find the beauty in stillness. If something happens, I am much more able to sit with it and see what happens rather than act straight away. I've learned that not everything needs a reaction, and many issues in life will resolve without getting worked up by them.

I've learned to discern the difference between discomfort and pain. By working with this in my yin practice, I have become more resilient. This ties back into learning to overcome my reactionary nature.

Through teaching this practice, I witness profound shifts in others. Students with real Type A personalities have over time softened their approach to their practice. I've also seen this transfer into the way they practice more yang styles as well. Instead of always going for the hardest possible option, I've seen them accept an invitation to listen to how they are feeling on a particular day and practice in accordance with those needs, rather than the need of the mind always wanting to be the 'best'.

Students of mine have shared with raw honesty how difficult they found a practice that they had perceived as easy because it was just sitting around in floor postures. When faced with stillness and quiet they've found it to be a challenge. I encourage them to stick with it and see what happens over time. Some do, some don't. I like to think that those that don't will return later.

Some students have told me that yin yoga is the only way they can meditate. The sensation in the body during the pose gives them something to focus on, rather than just sitting with thoughts and breath. Indeed, I recall my own teacher describing yin yoga as the gateway drug to meditation, and I totally agree!

Michelle, yin yoga teacher

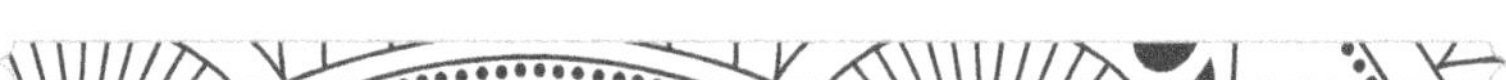

Wu Wei as an Aspect of Yin

Wu wei is the potion to soothe our yin deficit. Like yin, *wu wei* is the feminine. Moving with our own *wu wei* nature is what we may also call *'li'* which is a Chinese word that refers to organic pattern or grain, like the grain of wood. *Li* is the spiral of a snail shell, the pattern of marble, the sacred geometry of flowers. When we are moving with the flow, all is well and beautiful!

Stillness is healing and helpful. But to heal does not mean that we completely stop moving forever. It's rather about learning when (and how) to be still.

To truly heal, it's balance we are seeking. To come in line with *wu wei*, effortlessness of mind, is not necessarily an equal balance, but natural harmony, making a conscious choice about engaging with yang and engaging with yin. For example, we may spend one hour in a day engaged in force or control – enjoying a run or lifting heavy weights – but the rest of the day may be more easeful. We can really enjoy that forceful action when we are well-rested and calm of mind. And then we can enjoy returning to a more yin place once more. Yin is where our sustainable power source resides.

Yoga Equivalent

Wu wei could be compared to aparigraha – one of the yama in Patanjali's Eight Limbs of Yoga, which translates as 'non-grasping' 'non-greed' and 'non-attachment'. To accept each moment (and change) without either trying to cling too hard or reject it, but to accept and allow. Aparigraha is also one of the central teachings in the yogic text, The Bhagavad Gita, in which the character Krishna shares the lesson we explored earlier in this book: "Let your concern be with action alone, and never with the fruits of action. Do not let the results of action be your motive." It's not the destination, which is something we can sometimes get fixated on, but rather the journey that really matters.

PREPARING TO PRACTICE

If you are new to yin yoga, yoga in general or to practicing by yourself at home rather than in a class, you may have some practical questions. I offer the following as support and guidance.

Prepare your space: One of the beauties of yin yoga is that you can do it pretty much anywhere you have a little space to spread out! Find yourself somewhere lovely: the garden, a soft carpet, on your bed and create a simple sanctuary for yourself. Put your phone on silent. Get a blanket, and cushions or a bolster beside you. You might want them for support or warmth, and you might not, but it's useful to have them nearby. Extra delights might include lighting candles, incense or some soothing music if you like.

Timing: Read through the sequence to get a sense of the poses before you start. You can set a timer on your phone for a few minutes for each pose. People who already listen to my meditations on the awesome Insight Timer app might already know this; they have a great timer function so you can set a lovely chime to go off, say every three minutes for thirty minutes, which is excellent for yin yoga practice at home, or just settle in for a time that feels good. And of course, I have created videos for all the Yin Magic sequences, so do join me in video form on my website and I'll do all the serious stuff of counting!

With a timer, you'll be told when to change poses; but if you are feeling pain or pins and needles, bring yourself out gently whenever you feel the need. Moving between the poses should be slow and mindful. Muscles that have had a good long stretch and pause are weaker in strength than tight or active muscles, so take your time to move gently, pause, breath, wiggle gently if you need to.

In some yin classes, the teacher will guide you into a *savasana* between every pose as a kind of 'reset' button. I've not done that in my sequences but encourage you to take your time in your own way.

There is a trinity of 'rules' in yin yoga: three simple principles that give you an overview of what the practice is about:

1. Move into the pose to where you can feel the stretch (sometimes called the 'edge'): moving slowly and gently, never stretch so far as to cause pain.

2. Resolve to be still. Consciously try to release and settle into the pose.

3. Hold the pose for an extended period of time. This might be 1 or 2 minutes to begin with, progressing to 5 minutes or more.

Breathing: Taking an easeful breath is always a great way to start, as we arrive in our practice think about this journey to bring the body, breath and mind to a place of calm, of unhurriedness and of ease. Your whole being is slowing down in this yin journey. You might also like to try a simple *pranayama,* like a deep belly breath or three-part breath, where we inhale for three slow counts and then exhale for three, especially if we want to bring your awareness to the breath or the lungs.

Attention: We want our focus to be within, perhaps it's the area you are feeling a stretch, maybe it's your breath, maybe it's your connection to the earth, or noticing any emotions or sensations that arise.

Eating: Often hatha yoga classes will recommend leaving two or three hours after eating before practising, but because yin yoga is so slow, it may be you don't need so much of a gap. That being said, poses like twists and folds can be more enjoyable if you haven't just eaten a big bowl of spaghetti! So, give yourself at least an hour after eating a meal.

Contraindications

Contraindication is a word we use in yoga teaching for a reason not to practice a pose (or to ensure you do an adapted version) if you have a specific condition or injury. Part of yoga practice is an exploration with intention and attention. So treat each practice and each new pose as research in a way, developing your own sensitivity to what works and what doesn't. If you are unsure, it's always wise to check with your doctor first, and/or seek a yin yoga class where you can talk to your teacher.

Your intention is always to create space, stimulate the meridian lines and organs and connect to your body from a place of love. It is never to push yourself into pain, or feel that you need to force your body into any kind of pose – that's a rule for anyone coming to any form of yoga.

Here's a useful reminder:

We do not use the body to get into a pose –
we use the pose to get into our body.
Bernie Clarke

In yoga, it does not matter how far you stretch, it never has. So don't push, strain, struggle. Just allow yourself to be, to know, to listen – that's far more valuable than being 'flexible'. Stress inhibits the flow of *qi*, so it is essential that you do not push into pain: if you are not feeling safe or comfortable, you'll not receive the full benefits of the pose.

Do listen to your body: if you feel any tingling in the limbs like pins and needles, this can be a sign of nerve compression, which isn't damaging in the time frames we are using, but you'll want to slowly ease out of the pose, either taking the pose more gently or taking a break to relax, release the nerve and let blood flow. If you are coming to a yin class with nerve compression issues like sciatica, it can be a super helpful practice, so it is, as always, about balance and listening to the body.

Pregnancy: The standard advice is that you shouldn't start any new physical activity during pregnancy. If you have done some yoga before then yin should be fine. You may want to avoid twists or anything that feels like it's putting pressure on your belly (and avoid lying flat on the back in the final trimester). Explore Butterfly Pose and Child's Pose with wide knees, which should feel nice to gently open the hips, with plenty of space for the belly.

Postpartum: A gentle postpartum yoga routine can be wonderful to make time for yourself with gentle, soothing movement. Poses like Hanging Forward Fold, Shoelace and Child's Pose would be great places to start. Save twists and backbends only for when you feel ready. Listen to your body, and don't push yourself.

Menstruation: This will be down to your own listening, but I find yin is one of my favourite practices at this time because of its soothing, yin feminine nature. Sometimes when the belly feels delicate, twists and hip openers might feel uncomfortable, so bring in plenty of support if you need it. For example, in Reclining Butterfly Pose, bring a cushion or block under each knee. If you are feeling achy or crampy, bring in plenty of support and extra layers for warmth.

Low blood pressure: people with low blood pressure can experience dizziness and nausea when exercises involve sudden changes in posture – which makes yin yoga a good choice as we are moving slowly. It can also help blood circulation. Just be aware to move slowly when rising from any forward folds.

Hypermobility: With hypermobility, joints have an extreme/large range of movement. This can be caused by a variety of factors and can increase during pregnancy, postpartum and the pre-menstrual and menstrual phases of the cycle. If your hypermobility is due to conditions such as Ehlers Danlos Syndrome, seek your doctor's advice.

If you have hypermobility and want to try yin yoga, start easefully with shorter holds of one or two minutes, and don't take the pose to the very end of your range of motion. Bring in props for support. Take time to notice how you feel during and after the practice, and if you wish, work towards longer holds. Poses like Child's Pose, Waterfall and Easy Seat would be a good place to start.

Chronic Pain: If you suffer from chronic pain with conditions such as sciatica, fibromyalgia and/or ME, yoga can seem out of reach as a practice. But yin yoga offers a pathway to yoga and the potential for some pain relief.

Yin yoga can still be challenging, so if yin is too much, restorative yoga or yoga nidra might be for you. In restorative yoga, you do not hold deep stretches but instead surrender into relaxing poses, gently finding space in the body whilst supported by props. As the name suggests, this practice gives the body opportunity to heal and restore.

If in any doubt, please do seek a teacher who will be able to support and advise you on a personal basis.

ALCHEMY OF THE ELEMENTS - MAGICAL YIN YOGA SEQUENCE

Now we've explored the theoretical foundations of yin yoga and the practical preparations, let's get moving (slowly)!

I've taken some of the ideas of *wu xing* to weave together and inspire a yin practice, because for me this is really the crucible of where yin yoga, magic, alchemy can all combine into something special and wonderful, and at the same time deliciously easeful!

If you are inspired by the alchemical transformation through the elements, here is a yin sequence to support your journey. These are yin poses that connect to the energy of transformation and movement, the yin within the yang. From each element the next is born.

As we are seeking yin and grounding, I am starting and ending this sequence with the Earth element. I've brought in a few moving elements through this sequence that are not strictly yin – but which I feel embody the *wu xing* energy and help move *qi/prana* around the body.

You will find a video of this – and all of the sequences in the book – at sentiayoga.com/yinmagic

Earth: Child's Pose

It all begins with Earth, our mother. We are the child here. We find connection to the Earth meridian by sending arms reaching along the ground, gently opening through the front of body, tummy and heart space and connecting to the Earth's grounding energy.

Metal: Sphinx Pose

Strong and solid, Metal is drawn from the Earth. We rise like a golden sphinx gazing to the sun. From lying on your stomach, bring your forearms to the floor with your elbows under your shoulders, to raise your chest off the ground. Connection here is to the Lungs and Large Intestine meridians by opening through the front of the body, with a gentle back bend. Metal is the element of structure and boundaries. Be brave and set your boundaries, like a sphinx guarding the gates of your energy sources.

Water: Hanging Forward Fold

From standing, we are soft and easeful as we hang heavy through the upper body. Our connection here is to the Kidney and Bladder meridians by opening through the spine and hips and stretching the back of the legs.

Wood: Garland Pose

The torso and spine are, like the wood element, opening, blooming, growing tall in this low squat. Hands together in a prayer position, and extending through the spine. We explore the connection to the Liver and Gallbladder meridians by opening through the inner thighs. Wood, as an element, loves to rise, but we all need the flexibility to bend with the wind.

Fire: Easy Seated Flames

From cross-legged easy seat, we'll make flame movements with the arms and rolling hands, like a flamenco dancer. Then we'll take the arms out wide, flexing the hands with the fingers pointing up, so the hands make a 'stop' gesture. Then flex the wrists so the fingers point down. Take time with the movement and transformation and connect to the Heart meridian, by working through the shoulders and arms.

Easy seat fold

And then we return to Earth once more as we fold forwards. Returning to the Earth and the beginning of our cycle.

THE MAGIC OF STORY TIME

A good story is a powerful thing, not only to help us find the roots of our practices but also during our yoga journey on the mat.

Sutra means thread in Sanskrit, and the *Yoga Sutras* of Patanjali tell us a story about how to practice yoga, but also about drawing in our own threads of energy, attention and awareness that we send out into the world, encouraging us to explore our own inner threads a little closer.

The easeful, slow atmosphere and the attitude of acceptance present in yin yoga allow us to listen a little more deeply to the stories that are present in our lives and our relationships and work towards releasing the stories that no longer serve us, and the threads that bind us too tightly.

With yin yoga there is always time. Time to listen to our own story. Time to settle, to readjust, to start again from the beginning. Time to explore. Time to learn the appropriate depth in each posture. Time to attend, to notice, and to make mindful choices to reside in the here and now.

We can enjoy the gift of time that goes alongside stillness; precious time to get to know our body, what it needs and where our edges are. Some edges are physical, but we can also listen to and honour emotional and psychological edges in the alchemy of our practice – becoming a watcher of which stories rise and which stories fade.

We live in cultures that are constantly judging us. Are we good enough? Are we beautiful, smart or wealthy enough? And we know that the body is paying attention to every message that it's receiving. Trying always to be 'better' causes both physical and emotional stress. Yin yoga offers us a space for acceptance. When we bring a different attitude – that of compassion into our practice – our bodies respond in a very different way: we begin to accept ourselves. As we bring acceptance to our stories, our path of healing begins.

CLOSING YINSIGHTS

Yin yoga is an invitation to experience, feel and listen. In the yin postures, everything becomes an object of meditation. We feel our limits and take care of ourselves from moment to moment. This perspective may also help us to deal with feelings and sensations that arise in everyday life as we gain self-knowledge. We begin, finally, to hear our own story.

Within yin yoga, all postures are an invitation to stillness, to 'be' with yourself without judgement, and to work in harmony with your body. You may think of your body and energy in terms of organs and meridians, and how your practice may soothe these. Or maybe what you feel has no words, no titles, no lines or rules. The invitation is open!

4

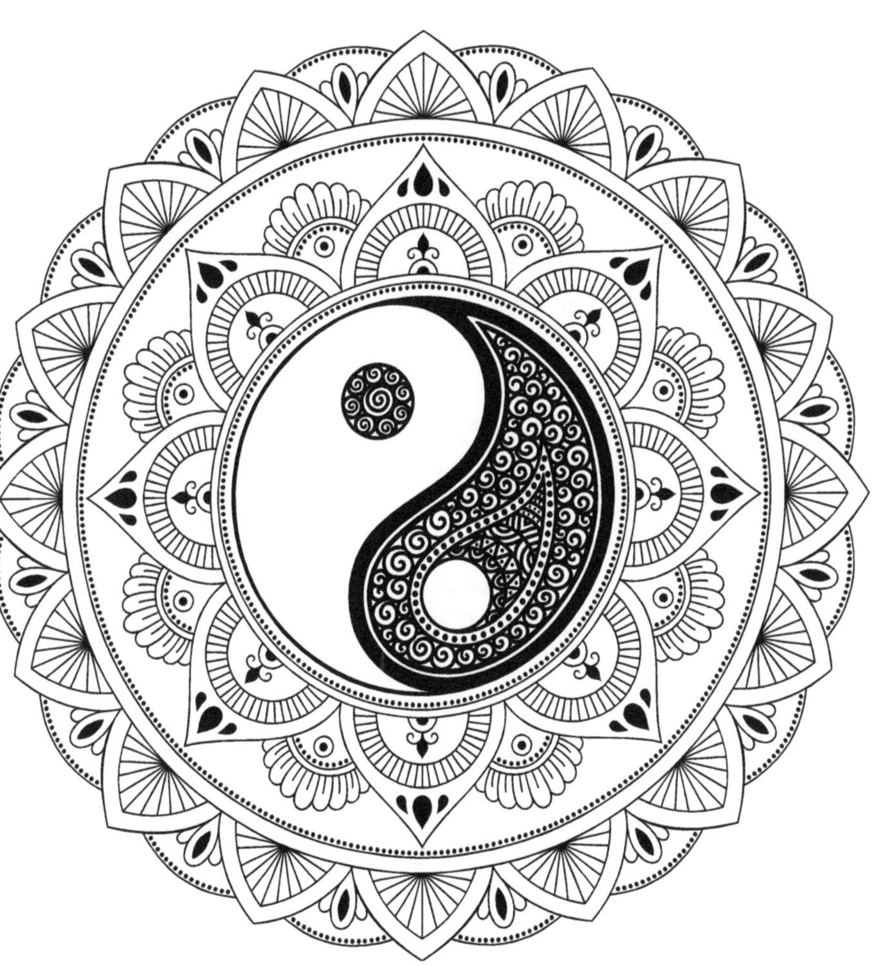

YIN ENERGY MEDICINE

As we have learned from the Tao – all things are energy.

Within the Chinese medicine tradition, the specific energies that work within us are understood to flow through meridians. The meridian system is a web of energy lines that connects the entire body together both physically and energetically. There are six major yin meridians and six yang meridians that link together the organs in the body, which we will explore in more detail in this chapter.

Using the meridian lines as a guide for yogic practice is unique to yin yoga, and can help us understand how yin yoga can access the energy that moves through the body. If you attend a yin yoga class the teacher will almost certainly mention the meridians, to explain the organs or energy we are connecting to in the pose, or in their connections to the *wu xing* elements or seasons.

This chapter will help you to understand a little more how yin yoga poses work with the meridians and organs. You do not need to know about this in order to enjoy yin yoga, but it can be nice to learn a little of the philosophy behind the practice, as it differs from the Western medical understanding of the body. Acupuncturists and doctors of Chinese medicine spend years learning the complex meridian maps of the body, so you won't become an expert overnight. And if this is too technical for your interests right now, feel free to skip ahead to the next chapter.

THE ORGANS

In Chinese medicine each organ and its connected meridian have their own physiological and energy functions. When written down they are usually capitalised to illustrate that. So, for example Heart, is used to reference the meridian, energy and emotional systems connected to the heart, as opposed to simply the heart as an individual physical organ in the way that it is understood within the Western medical tradition.

The main yin organs are the Liver, Spleen, Heart, Lungs and Kidneys.

The yang organs are Gallbladder, Stomach, Small Intestine, Large Intestine and Bladder.

Each of these organs are connected to the five elements and the meridians share the same element so, for example, the Kidney organ and the Kidney meridian are both Water. In addition to their structure and functions, organs are also linked to emotional and energetic well-being. As long as *qi* can flow freely through your meridians and your organs, your body will be harmonious and healthy. But imbalance or blocks can occur through stress or trauma. This affects the function of the organ connected to the blocked meridian and ultimately, your whole being.

Pairings

The major organs are connected via meridian lines in yin and yang pairs. For example, Lungs (yin) form a pair with the Large Intestine (yang). Each pairing is also connected to a particular element and emotion. The yin and the yang organs are part of one system, so if one of them is out of balance, it will affect its counterpart as well.

We may work directly with the organs or with particular physical or emotional blocks through the meridians. For instance, if you are feeling a lot of anger and frustration, you may have an excess of fire *qi*, and you may work with your Water-Kidney meridian through specific yin yoga pose to release or 'wash away' this intense emotion and return to balance. Too much yang energy in the Stomach/Spleen could be felt as anxiety or tummy ache, a yin yoga practice with a focus on the Stomach, like gentle twists, could help soothe this excess of yang.

Emotional imbalances can be addressed through yin yoga practice, which in turn can soothe physiological imbalances – our emotions are rooted in our organs, and our organs affect our emotions – it's a cycle. And yoga connects to bring harmony to the whole being – body, mind and soul.

YIN	YANG
Kidneys	**Bladder**
Water Element: associated with moisture and flowing.	
Emotional pairing: Fear/Wisdom.	
Liver	**Gallbladder**
Wood Element: germination, extension, softness and harmony.	
Emotional pairing: Anger/Creativity.	
Heart	**Small Intestine**
Fire Element: aspects of heat, expansion, and transformation.	
Emotional pairing: Agitation or Overwhelm/Joy.	
Lungs	**Large Intestine**
Metal Element: cleansing, removing, strength and firmness.	
Emotional pairing: Sadness/Gratitude.	
Spleen	**Stomach**
Earth Element: aspects of transformation, growth and nourishment.	
Emotional pairing: Anxiety/Compassion.	

The Sixth Pair

The eagle-eyed among you will have noticed that there are only five organs in this table. That is because the sixth pairing – the Pericardium and Triple Burner/Triple Warmer – is a little different, as neither are physical organs of the body. They are paired together under the Fire element. (Fire being the only element which governs two pairs of organs – Heart and Small Intestine being the other.)

The pericardium is a protective tissue that lines the heart. The Pericardium meridian is a yin meridian, descending through the diaphragm and the abdomen where it connects with the Triple Burner meridian.

The Triple Burner meridian is yang; its general function being warming and energy, but also a way of grouping together parts of the body. It doesn't exist in the physical sense, as is the case with the other organs/tissues. The Triple Burner moves and marshals resources in the body, and in modern Western medicine might be seen as comparable to the immune system. The three burning 'spaces' of the triple burner are:

- The Upper Burner from the neck to the diaphragm, connected to the breath.
- The Middle Burner, which is connected to the digestive process.
- The Lower Burner is responsible for discharging bodily waste.

I wanted to mention them here, so as not to miss them off the list, but I will be grouping the Pericardium with the Heart for practices to open the heart space and the Fire element – and we'll explore the Triple Burner/*tan tien* cauldrons more in the next chapter.

MAPPING THE MERIDIANS

The meridian maps of the body are beautiful and complex, but I don't want to overwhelm you with too much technical information here. So I'll just give you a basic outline of some of the influences of meridians and organs within the body within this philosophy. And we'll get to know the meridians a little more when we start exploring yoga poses later in this chapter.

You can find more meridian maps at sentiayoga.com/yinmagic and in the books I've outlined in the reading list at the end of the book.

On this map, you'll also see the governor and conception vessels that run up through the centreline of the body. They are known as vessels rather than meridians as energy can be held here like reservoirs and dispersed through the body/meridians when needed. The Conception Vessel is rather beautifully known as the 'Sea of Yin' and Governor as the 'Sea of Yang'. Practices such as *pranayama* and meditation can help nourish these seas.

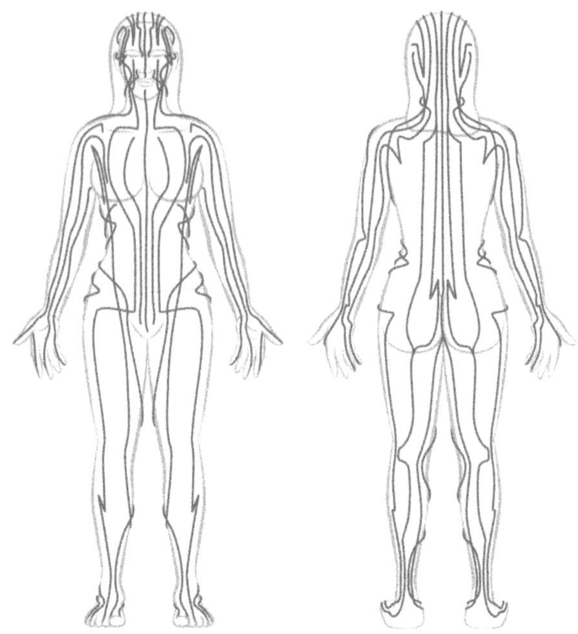

Meridian of the Kidney/Bladder

The Kidney area is also known as the 'Root of Life'. The kidneys are a strong power source, a source of essential energy, as they include the adrenal glands. The Kidney meridian is the energy line that leads all the others. Starting at the sole of the foot, running up the inner leg until it reaches the kidneys and branches off to the bladder – its yang counterpart – and then rises up through the chest.

Meridian of the Liver/Gallbladder

The Liver meridian runs from the big toe up to the abdomen where it connects to the liver organ and Gallbladder. Corresponding with Wood energy, the liver and its meridian govern growth and development, ambitions and creativity.

Meridian of the Heart/Small Intestines

The Heart is known as the 'Emperor' of the organs, as it is thought to command all of the organs and viscera. The pericardium, the fascial lining around the heart muscle, holds the heart like a guardian or gatekeeper, providing an extra layer of protection. The Heart meridian starts at the heart organ and then branches out to the Small Intestine – its yang organ pair – as well as in routes through the chest and lungs.

Meridian of the Lungs/Large Intestine

The Lungs govern breath and energy and support the heart with the circulation of blood. The Lung meridian travels through shoulders, arms and hands. If energy cannot move freely through the Lungs and their meridian this may manifest as shortness of breath. This relationship between breath and pulse is the basis of Chinese breathing exercises, as well as many yogic *pranayama* techniques: our connection of yoga and breathwork helps us move *qi/prana* around the body.

Meridian of the Spleen/Stomach

The Spleen meridian represents the Earth element. The Spleen/Stomach pairing are connected to energy of compassion. The Spleen meridian runs from the big toe, running up through to the stomach and then to the chest, heart and throat. Symptoms of disharmony in the Spleen/Stomach line can include anxiety and stomach problems.

YIN YOGA SEQUENCES FOR THE MERIDIANS

Yin yoga helps balance internal organs by gently stimulating them and their associated meridians, helping the energy of that organ to flow freely, bringing organs back into a state of wellbeing. So, for these sequences ahead, I'm using the yin organs and meridian of Heart/Pericardium, Lungs, Spleen, Liver and Kidneys to assist us in cultivating and nourishing our yin nature.

YIN POSES FOR THE HEART MERIDIAN

Yin poses that connect to the Heart are those that target the upper inner arms, shoulders and heart space.

Heart Melting Pose

This pose is a nice backbend for the upper and mid-back. It also opens through the shoulders, chest and armpits, areas the Heart meridian travels through.

From hands and knees, walk your hands forward, allowing the chest to open down towards the floor. Keep the hips stacked above your knees. You can soften the arms, so your elbows rest on the earth, forehead or chest can also rest upon the earth.

Child's Pose

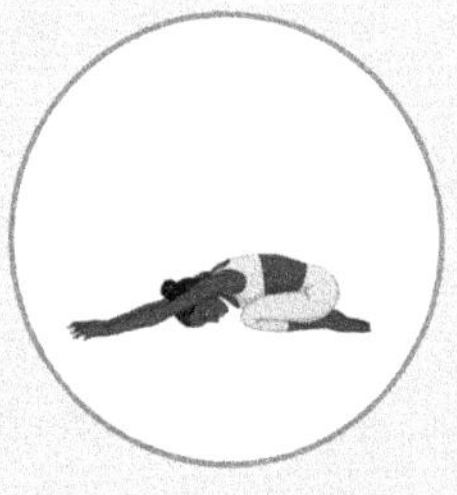

From all fours sit your bum back on your heels, take the knees out a little wider than the hips. Your forehead can rest upon the earth and arms reach easefully towards the top of your mat. This is our Child's Pose, and we can settle here.

Reclining Twist

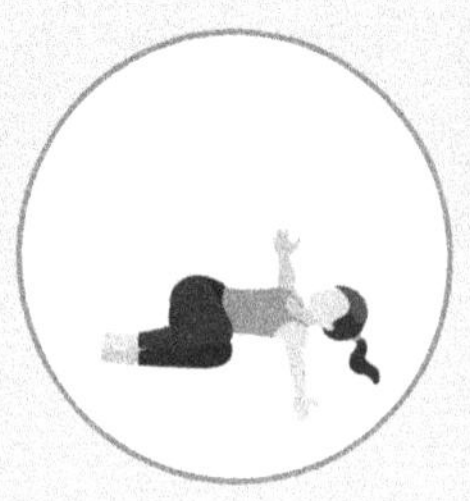

Lying down on your back, place the soles of the feet on the ground. Open your arms wide on the earth and let the knees fall to the left side, the head can gaze to the right. Repeat on both sides.

The Magic of Twists

Whilst stretching any muscle releases serotonin (the brain's happy chemical) into the bloodstream, twists are an especially great way to soothe and nurture harmony in the body. The twisting motion helps massage the digestive organs, encouraging *qi* to flow smoothly in the Small Intestine (the yang organ paired with the yin Heart).

Spinal twists also gently stimulate the vagus nerve. Much of the information of the calming, parasympathetic nervous system travels through this nerve, which runs from the skull down the spine, supporting the regulation of the heart, lungs, and digestive system.

YIN POSTURES FOR THE LUNG MERIDIAN

Breathing can affect the nervous system; this relationship is the basis for breathwork and meditation in yoga. Conscious breathing creates a bridge between body and mind. By working with the lungs and breath in our practice, we can work towards bringing both to harmony.

Yin poses for the Lungs/Large Intestine meridians are those that open the upper body and the inner arms, similar to those for the Heart meridian. So, you could use the Heart Melting Pose and Reclining Twist that you learned above, as well as these next ideas.

Fish

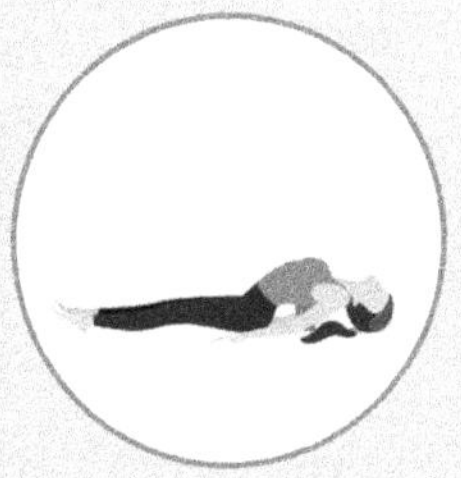

This is a gorgeous opener for the Heart and Lungs. From lying flat on your back, bring a bolster or cushion under the upper back to allow the opening of the front of your body. Your head can be supported or you can let it fall back a little to open through the throat. The arms can be resting above the head or by the hips. Legs can be straight or bring the soles together as in Butterfly (p66).

Bananasana

This name is a little play on the Sanskrit names that more traditional yoga poses have.

I make the same 'joke' every single time I guide my students into this pose, poor things, they must be sick of it by now! I say the official name of this pose is the Banana, but that's very unromantic, so I call it the Crescent Moon. I tell my students they can imagine they are a banana if they like, or a crescent moon, whichever brings them most calm!

Lying on your back take your arms above your head and carry your hands over to the right top corner of your mat and feet to the bottom right, so you create a crescent shape with your hips and shoulders still on the ground. (The icon here shows the image as seen from above.)

YIN POSTURES FOR THE SPLEEN MERIDIAN

Yin poses that help attend to the Spleen meridian are those that target the feet, legs and hips: our connection to the earth.

Lizard

Start on your hands and knees. Step your left foot to the ground outside your left hand. Bring this foot forward until the knee is above the ankle. Slide the right knee backward as far as you can. You may keep your hands on the ground or come to elbows (as pictured). Bring in the support of a blanket or cushion under the back knee if needed.

Swan

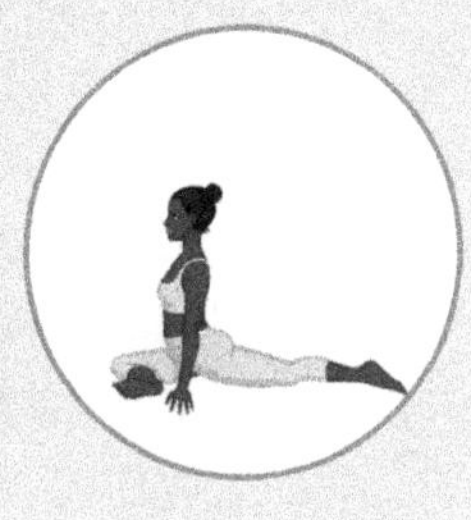

The Swan provides the quadriceps and hip flexors a stretch with a deep external rotation in the front of the hip. (known to Hatha Yogis as the Pigeon Pose)

Come into the pose from hands and knees. Slide your right knee behind your right wrist. To increase the intensity, bring the right foot forward, towards the left wrist, keeping the foot flexed – so your lower leg is crossing the centre line of the mat. If the sensation in the knee is too much, bring the right foot closer toward the left hip.

We are aiming to keep the hips square, so bring support in the form of a block or bolster under the right hip, if needed. Slide the left leg away behind you to open hips towards the earth. From here you can stay supported on hands or melt the body down onto forearms or rest on the earth (known as Sleeping Swan).

Toe Stretch

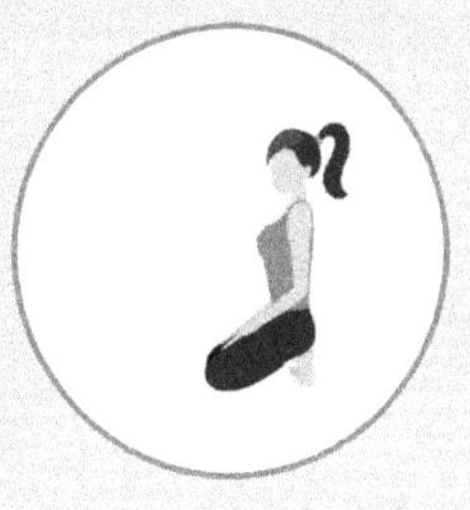

We spend about a minute in this pose in my classes, and that's usually challenging enough! From all fours; tuck the toes under and then sit back on the heels with the spine vertical, so the body's weight is helping stretch out the soles of the feet. Breathe. Stay here for two minutes at most. And take some nice tippy taps to release!

YIN POSTURES FOR THE LIVER MERIDIAN

These are three easeful poses that target the area of the inner legs and hips, to help restore Liver imbalances and to find a softness and harmony within the body.

Butterfly

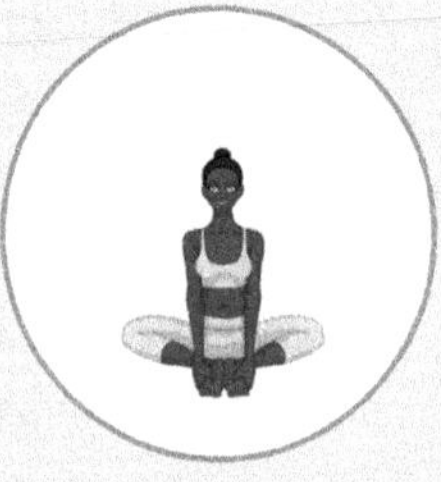

From Easy Seat, put the soles of your feet together, drawing your heels towards your hips. Hinging forward into a fold, rest your hands on your feet or the floor in front of you. Let your head hang heavy.

Dragonfly

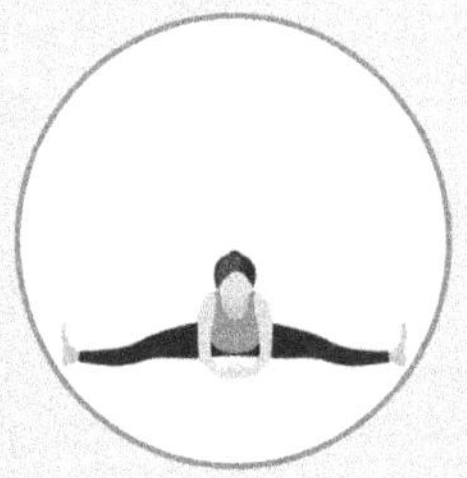

Bring yourself to a wide-legged seated position. You'll feel a stretch along the inner thighs with your hands placed in front of you as you hinge forward from the hips. Sitting on a cushion can help tilt the hips forward. Feel free to rest your arms on a bolster or cushion, let your head and neck be soft as you find calm.

Happy Baby

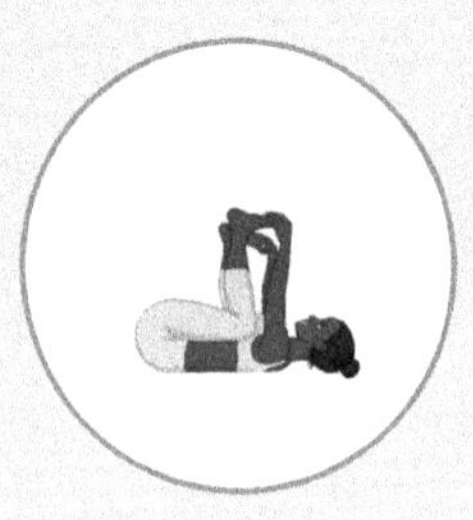

Lying on your back, hug knees to your chest. Draw your knees wide towards your armpits, and shine your soles to the ceiling, taking hold of the outer edges of the feet. Relax your head and shoulders on the floor.

If this feels too much, you can do Half Happy Baby, holding onto the knees, drawing them in toward your armpits.

YIN POSTURES FOR THE KIDNEY MERIDIAN

Yin poses that help connect to the Kidney meridian target the back and spine. In connecting to the Kidney and its partner the Bladder we are connecting to the Water element of the body, cooling excess heat and calming the mind – useful if you are feeling very yang or overly fiery.

Sphinx

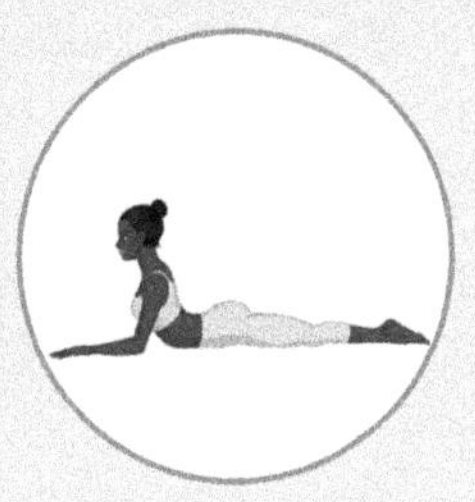

Start off by lying on your stomach. Bring your forearms to the floor with your elbows under your shoulders, to raise your chest off the ground. Notice how this feels in your lower back and gently engage your core muscles by drawing your tummy button toward your spine, to support your lumbar spine. Extend your legs along the ground behind you to gently anchor to the earth.

Snail

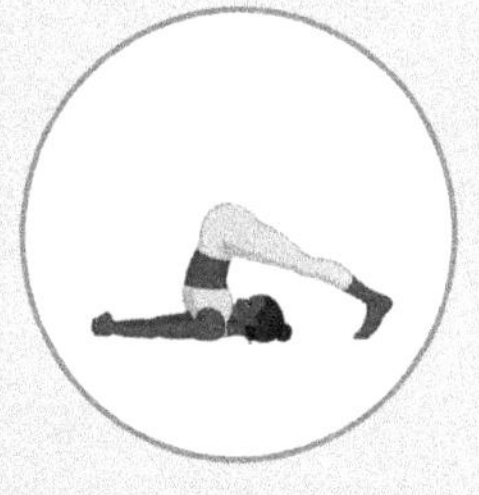

Start by lying on your back. Lift your hips, supporting them with your hands, draw your knees towards your face. Allow your back to round and gently lengthen the legs to bring your feet towards the floor above your head. The weight of your body will shift more onto your shoulders. If your legs are touching the floor, your hands can come to the floor behind the back.

If your feet do not touch the ground, you can do the pose close to a wall and place your feet on the wall, or onto a cushion or block.

Garland

In this squat, your feet are rooted into the ground. With your feet a little wider than your hips, drop into a low squat. You can use your hands to steady yourself or bring your palms together and hold them close to your heart centre in prayer. The Garland Pose also connects to the Bladder meridian, which runs down the back of the body, through the spine. And both kidney and bladder meridians journey through the legs.

CLOSING YINSIGHTS

We could view our whole physical body as yin, and the bustling life within it as yang. To hold the body in yin, allows some of those multiple yangs – busy mind, scattered thoughts, stresses, worries, tensions, ideas – to release. As we come back to our foundations, the constants of our being; body and bones, bringing more awareness to the energy that moves through us, the life that moves through us, allows magic, in its many forms, to move through us as well. As energy runs through our body, life runs through our body. Frameworks such as the meridians offer us a map and a guide, a structure with which to visualise this inner flow. The seas and rivers of energy flow through us and we can work towards nourishing and guiding a smooth watercourse. We can help this energy flow, through calming and opening the body (with yoga asana) mind (with meditation and mindful awareness) and breath (with *pranayama*).

5

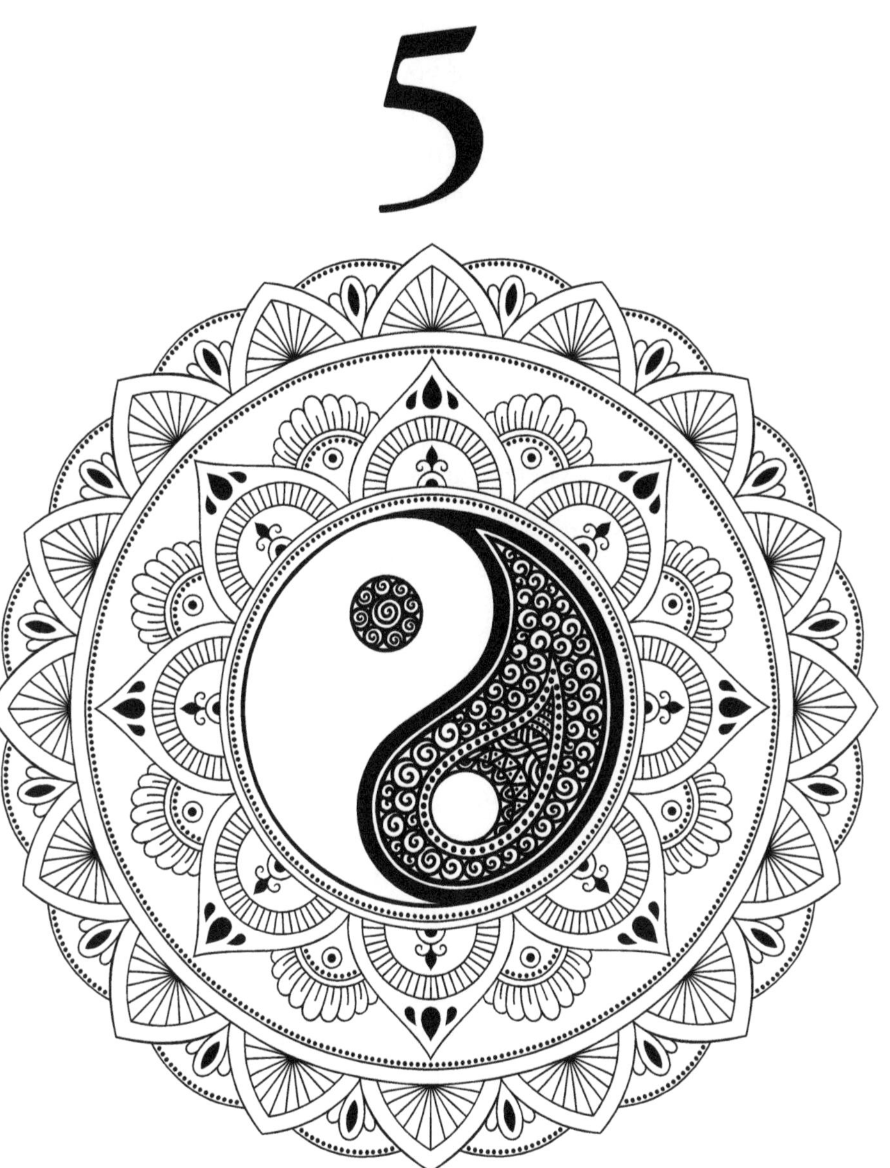

YIN ALCHEMY

If you search the internet for yin magic, you'll find some lovely articles about the 'magic' of yin yoga, in the sense that it is a beneficial practice. This is very true: there is abundant magic to be found in the process of doing this form of yoga, and of using yin yoga to access stillness and compassion.

But I am excited to shine more light onto the topic of the magical history and theology behind yin as a premise, drawn from Chinese culture with a rich history of magical practice including alchemy, sorcery and witchcraft. I want to highlight the fact that yin yoga has taken an element of a highly magical culture and history... and celebrate that in the hopes that it will enhance your practice of yin yoga, magic and embracing yin in your day.

The Power of The Way

Taoism is so full of magic I could write a whole book on the subject (but luckily for us, more expert authors have done just that. Check out the Reading List to learn more!). So here I will try and keep my exploration of the magic, sorcery and alchemy of Taoism under the topic of our exploration of yin.

The roots of Taoist magic trace all the way back to Neolithic times when shamans and wise men created writing as a form of magic – much like the ancient Egyptians who revered the magic and power within each written word.

Then as culture moved into the period of the dynasties, alchemy grew slowly into a popular form of magic as kings and influential men sought immortality, knowledge and power. The practice of Taoist magic invokes and channels the powers of the natural elements for health, wealth and prosperity. Techniques these ancient practitioners explored for achieving immortality included diet, herbs, breath control, meditation and the use of magical talismans.

By the Qin dynasty in China (221 to 206 BCE) Taoist magic flourished. Alchemists and magicians sought for themselves (and often their royal benefactors) connection with the Tao in order to obtain its mystical power, which transcends all earthly troubles... and maybe even death.

Energy Magic

In my previous book, Yoga for Witches, I shared the following words on energy magic, which I want to return to here, if the idea of energy magic is new to you.

"What we are doing in yoga and witchcraft is connecting to our inner power in our own depths and learning to harness the energies around us too. The energies that flow within and around the body affect us in physical, emotional and spiritual ways. This energy is often referred to as qi in Chinese traditions and prana in Indian traditions. As a witch, you may call this energy magic."

TAOIST ALCHEMY

Alchemy is, simply put, a process of transformation: it may be symbolically, psychologically, or magically. It was present in some form in many Eastern and Western cultures, as an ancient forerunner of modern-day sciences like chemistry. Alchemy is a process of taking something ordinary, and from it creating something extraordinary, sometimes in ways that cannot be explained by traditional science, hence it is often considered a magical practice.

Inner alchemy *(neidan)* and outer alchemy *(waidan)* are part of an array of spiritual practices that make up Taoist alchemy, intended to lengthen life and create forms of immortality. Tao alchemists sought a *jindan* "golden elixir", indeed, their tradition was often known as The Way of the Golden Elixir *(jindan zhi tao)*. Chinese medicine is a descendant of these ancient alchemical creations of herbal elixirs for health and longevity.

Whilst Eastern alchemy has always been focused on the golden elixir of immortality, as the practice swept over to the West, the goal transformed itself in many practices into seeking gold of a solid metal nature, turning base metals into gold. I think this is a fascinating reflection on these cultures and how they value time and money differently!

External alchemy *(waidan)* covers ceremonial magic and rituals, and the world beyond our own physical body, much like the work of the priestesses and oracles of ancient Greece and Rome. External alchemists would explore knowledge towards one's relationship with society and the physical environment, seeking insight into the spirit world and universe, and the development of psychic and superhuman abilities (just like the Siddhis of Hindu culture).

Ceremonial Taoist magic holds many similarities with Pagan and Druid culture, such as calling on the four directions, the use of herbs in potions, and runes and sigil work for manifestation and divination.

Internal alchemy *(neidan)* is a practice that seeks harmony and good health. As the name suggests, inner alchemy is inner work: the relationships within oneself, body mind and spirit – discernment of one's inner divinity (and demons). Meditation and mantra would be popular tools just as in Buddhist and yogic traditions.

Much like the many ways one may explore witchcraft and magic, the study and purpose of both *waidan* and *neidan* were to explore the mystical and the magical, but from different viewpoints. In meditation, for example, like the trances and spiritual journeys of magicians, shamans, oracles and hedgewitches, the Taoist mystic would visualise gods that inhabit the human body *(neidan)* and as they occupy the universe *(waidan)*. With divination they would focus both on seeing the pattern of life in practices such as the study of stars and on discerning patterns of the earth as portents for our own personal lives *(neidan)* as well as that of the world and society *(waidan)*.

In both Eastern and Western traditions, alchemists sought to create potions that bestowed immortality and to attain life-prolonging energy through spiritual purification. Within this idea of prolonging life, you could definitely draw in our ideas of yin and seeking stillness. We know very well in the West that chronic stress and lack of attention to wellness can shorten lives and foster 'dis-ease'. So, in our own way, by finding calm, we are bringing just a little of that golden elixir to our own being, to live long and happy lives, and to savour each day.

Alchemy and Transformation in Western Psychology

Carl Gustav Jung (a student and collaborator of Sigmund Freud's in the early twentieth century, and the founder of analytical psychology) spent much of his life studying alchemy and spirituality in relation to the nature of the human psyche. This, he thought, could only be understood with symbols and archetypes that are able to contain our paradoxes and ambiguities. To him, alchemy reflected the process of personal transformation in the metaphor of alchemists moulding base metals into gold. (Though intrigued by many aspects of Eastern cultures, especially mandalas, as a European he draws on Western ideas of alchemy). Jung suggested that feelings can be purified and integrated in much the same way as the alchemical process, allowing us to see ourselves and our world from a deeper perspective.

His approach to internal alchemy was expressed as seven stages of transformation. Originally used in relation to the chemical transformations of alchemy, you will notice how they can be equated to personal transformation. Though our personal experience might not perfectly match up with all these stages, it is a useful framework to the invisible journey through the layers of our psyche towards what Jung called individuation: a mindful awareness of who you are in the world.

The first stage is **Calcination**, the heating. A traumatic event or a build-up of challenges may act as a catalyst for the cycle of transformation to begin. We may also initiate the process through our own determination to explore and uncover old ways of being that hold us back.

The second stage is **Solution**, like the dissolving of substances in water after the fire has burnt through the old structures. After the burning away and dissolving – what's left?

Next comes **Coagulation**, a solidifying of what remains. We can begin to explore and accept edges and boundaries as we find a way of coming back together.

In this process of coming back together we reach **Sublimation**, which is a dissipation of energy. We have to get clearer still on where we want to direct our energy and what now needs to be let go.

The 'letting go' makes up the next stage, **Mortification**, a death of sorts. This shedding and stepping out of our old skin is the next stage of **Separation**.

The final stage of the cycle, **Conjunction**, is union: just as we seek in yoga! This culmination of the process allows us to integrate the parts of us that remain and fully embody them.

What is interesting is that what at first appears to be a negative and destructive process, a breakdown – something we have been taught to avoid – is actually a highly creative and fruitful one. Though we can add our conscious effort and awareness, the process is very yin, it happens in the dark of our unconscious minds. This is another lesson in the magic of yin: that what cannot be seen or consciously controlled is just as powerful, if not more so, than that which we visibly control with effort.

THE THREE TREASURES

From Tao arises one; from one arises two; from two arises three and from three arise the ten thousand things.

Lao Tzu

We have explored the Tao and the one *qi*, the two being yin and yang, now let us explore the three…

The idea of *san bao* – Three Jewels or Treasures – is central to both internal and external Taoist alchemy, and has several representations within Chinese culture.

The Three Jewels of Chinese Buddhism refer to Buddha, Dharma, and Sangha. In Taoism, Three Treasures are the attributes of compassion, frugality and humility. And the Three Treasures of the body in Chinese medicine and alchemy are *jing*, *qi* and *shen* energy.

Is Three Really a Magic Number?

The number three is symbolic in Taoism, and we see it present in many other wisdom cultures as well: the image of the triple goddess, the holy trinity, the Celtic triskele... There are echoes of the power within the number three the world over. This tripartite understanding of human existence, of three energies or strands of the body that are woven together, comes through again and again in so many cultures.

Triads – groups of three people, things, or traits, are found in many concepts of the divine and spiritual. So abundant is this idea that I could take a whole chapter to list them all!

But why? Why is it so powerful? Who was first to do it? What does it mean?

There are many theories, and as with many ancient ideas, there is more than one answer. Triadic concepts can be traced back through the ancient world and the human connection to this number is strong enough to have been carried through worldwide cultures since ancient times. Throughout history, the number three has seemingly always had a unique significance. (However, I should also note that this is just one way of grouping together deities in ancient texts, other numbers do feature!) The following accounts are somewhat selective but do show some common patterns that are worth noting.

Indian

The *Rig Veda* (approx. 1100 BCE) feature threefold deities: Surya (sun), Vata (wind) and Agni (fire).

Another yogic text the *Upanishads* (approx. 800 BCE) refer to three *gunas*: qualities that characterise all living beings, which are harmony *(sattva)*, action *(rajas)*, and inertia *(tamas)*. The Trimurti is the triple deity of supreme divinity in Hinduism: Brahma the creator, Vishnu the preserver, and Shiva the destroyer.

Ancient Greek

Ancient Greek mythology has a profusion of triads: the rulers Hades, Poseidon and Zeus. The triple form of the goddess Hecate. The three-headed Cerberus. The Gorgons, the Charities, the Furies and the Fates all came in threes in various tales.

The Greek philosopher, Pythagoras (who lived around 500 BCE), proposed that the meaning behind numbers was deeply significant. For him, the number three represented harmony, wisdom and understanding. It was also the number of time – past, present, future; birth, life, death; beginning, middle, end. He is best remembered for the theorem that school children are still taught today – for three-sided shapes: triangles.

Buddhist

To the Buddhist the Three Jewels that support the path of living with awareness are:

Buddha – A reminder of our own divinity, inner radiance; the Buddha, our greatest teacher, is within us.

Dharma – Our natures' true calling and the path to refine our Buddha within.

Sangha – Our teachers, inspirations and connections.

Christian

In Christianity God is presented as Trinity: Father, Son and Holy Spirit. And how many Kings visited the baby Jesus? That's right… three!

Numerologists recognise that three is the number of the child – it symbolises growth and magic born from the combination of two other things: a metaphorical progeny brought forth from two parents, full of energy and possibility.

That rounds up nicely this journey with the number three – it presents a connection to energy and possibility. So let's get to our threes in Chinese, Tao and… Celtic cultures.

Taoist internal alchemy focuses upon transforming and balancing essential energies of the body sustaining human life, known as the three treasures, *san bao: jing*, the essence; *qi*, the life force and *shen*, the spirit.

These three energies unite within the cauldrons or crucibles of the body known as the *tan tien*. These are energy centres that hold the three *san bao* treasures: a very similar premise to that of the chakras as key points of *prana* energy. The main difference being that the Taoist *tan tien* are more about storing and transforming energy within the cauldrons – whereas the yogic chakras are more like gateways or vortices. *Tan tien* and the chakras may be separate, but they can certainly be cooperative energetic centres.

The three cauldrons are located within the body at the pelvis/belly, solar plexus/heart and head. Within them *jing*, *qi* and *shen* can be drawn in, stored and sent out into the rest of the body. These cauldrons might be considered yin holding in various ways the energy of *jing*, *qi*, and *shen* energy.

Lower ***tan tien (xia tan tien)***: This is located at the lower belly. Here you draw in *qi* energy (such as through meditation). The *qi* energy you are drawing in and your own innate *jing* energy can come together in this cauldron like ingredients of a potion – and together nurture new energy for your body and wellbeing. The lower *tan tien* corresponds to the yogic concept of the sacral *swadhisthana* chakra (which translates from Sanskrit to "home of self").

In Taoist meditation, much attention is devoted to connecting with the lower *tan tien* as it allows us to be physically and mentally rooted or 'grounded'. It is integral for yoga, spellwork and our journey to stillness.

Middle ***tan tien (zhong tan tien)***: Located at the heart, this cauldron is where *qi* is cultivated into *shen* spirit that then travels upwards. Also at this cauldron, the energy we draw in though the lungs and stomach is gathered and converted into *qi* that the body can use.

Upper ***tan tien (shang tan tien)***: Located at the head. Within this cauldron *shen* energy is refined into awareness, connection and consciousness, and *qi* is drawn on by the brain for focus and thought.

Three Crucibles in External Alchemy

In external alchemy *(waidan)*, the alchemy of ceremonial and ritual work, alchemists thought of this trio of cauldrons as being representative of the external elements that would need to be present and respected in any ceremonial work:

- ☾ Earth – Acknowledgement of earth and the natural world, such as calling in the four directions or honouring the seasons. We also see rituals honouring the natural world in Pagan, Wiccan and Hindu practices (to name just a few).
- ☾ Human – Your personal intentions, words and actions that need to be present and mindful in ritual.
- ☾ Heaven – A consideration of astrology includes stars, moon, sun, and deities, so a ceremony may be performed on an auspicious day, or under a certain lunar phase.

Cauldrons

Cauldrons are obviously a key symbol and tool of witchcraft and of Western alchemists. They are the container within which the magic of transformation occurs – literally and metaphysically.
Now perhaps you can also see that cauldrons have a significance in Chinese alchemy as well.
Almost all cauldrons in both East and West have three legs to represent the sacred number three (and also, to be fair, for the practical reason that three legs are more stable on an uneven surface!)
In Chinese magic, spellwork in cauldrons would have to acknowledge these three elements, a nod to law of trinities to ensure the harmony and balance and ultimate success of the spell. This is reflected in Western spellwork as well: a spell is often repeated three times, or multiples of threes are used (such as the nine knots of the Witch's Ladder).

CELTIC CAULDRONS

If you feel that this story of three cauldrons is familiar from a little closer to the West, you'd be right! A very similar idea exists in Celtic culture. In fact, there are some amazing similarities between Celtic and Chinese beliefs, as well as connections to the chakra lore of yogis.

Ancient Celtic texts describe the body as containing Three Cauldrons. These Three Celtic Cauldrons are the *Coire Goiriath* (Cauldron of Warming), the *Coire Ernmae* (Cauldron of Vocation), and the *Coire Sois* (Cauldron of Wisdom). Each of the Celtic Cauldrons is said to be connected through the inner fire and thread of connection which to many who follow Celtic lore may visualise as Brigid, Goddess of Fire: the home, hearth and forge. In this telling Goddess Brigid is the fire element, the element that transforms and ignites.

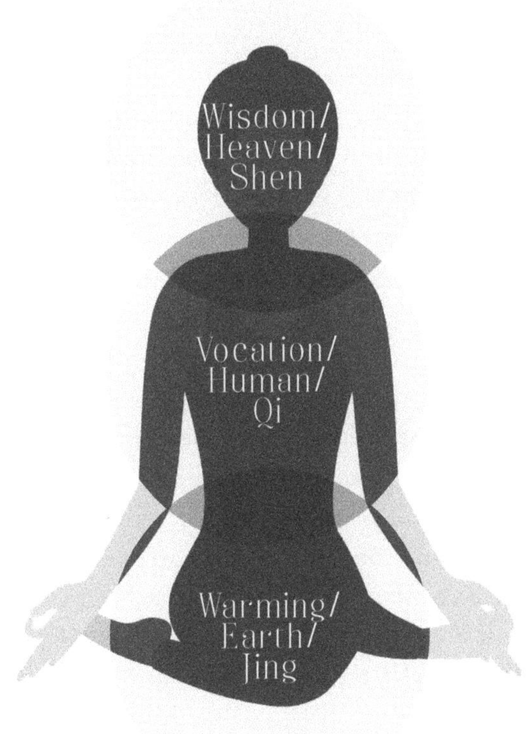

In both Chinese and Celtic traditions, we are presented with a representation of three essential elements to our wellbeing, grouped into three bodily areas, associated with cauldrons.:

Lower – Our sense of security and safety from our root, warming and connection to the earth.

Mid – Our ability to draw in nourishment in all its forms through the heart, stomach and lungs.

Upper – Our ability to think, to know, to make decisions and be inspired through the head and mind.

As well as the Three Cauldrons detailed below, there are also other significant cauldrons in Celtic myth that belong to the gods, and again we are presented with this idea that energy cauldrons may exist both within and outside of the body just as practitioners of *neidan* and *waidan* thought. Witches may well be familiar with the Cauldron of Knowledge owned by the goddess Kerridwen, who we'll meet in Chapter 9.

The Cauldron of Warming

The Cauldron of Warming is the cauldron of life, located within the areas of the belly, hips and pelvis. We are born with this cauldron upright, and it represents the fires of emotion, vitality and power. It contains the basic energy and wisdom we need to live, breathe, and grow. A yogi may compare this cauldron to the sacral, root and solar plexus chakras.

The Cauldron of Vocation

The Cauldron of Vocation is located in the heart and chest space. The Cauldron of Vocation represents the connection between the self and the energy of land, inner guidance and intuition. I see this as your space for igniting your inner drives and purpose, what a yogi would call our dharma. As we find our path and connect to our life's purpose, the cauldron fills. A yogi may also associate this cauldron with the heart and throat chakras, connected to love and truth.

The Cauldron of Wisdom

Found at the head, the Cauldron of Wisdom is thought to be upside down and empty in a person at birth. A person might spend an entire lifetime filling it with wisdom and knowledge. This cauldron rules our spiritual development, helping us to see connections between ourselves, our paths, the gods, and one another (just like... *shen!* Oh my stars, everything is connected, we are all one giant magical family!) This is also very similar to the crown and third eye chakras from yogic thought.

Inner Cauldron Work

Isn't this amazing, how these cultures from all corners of the earth have records of this idea of cauldrons within the body? And the fact that the cauldron is a common symbol of the witch. Just as I weave together yoga and witchcraft, I believe ideas such as that of the Three Cauldrons can also be woven together in thought and practice through cultures and religions.

The Three Cauldrons represent ideas of holding the energies of our physical wellbeing and groundedness, our emotional depth and resilience, and our creative and spiritual inspiration, a yin touchstone in today's chaotic world. Just as chakras can be imbalanced and exhibit negative traits, the Three Cauldrons can offer their own challenges, blocks and imbalances, but also provide us with a framework to seek alignment.

How can you fill your cauldrons with joy, hope and peace? How can you prevent others from slurping from these containers or stop following paths that stab holes in them, letting our energy drain out like water?

Activity: Cauldrons of Transformation

Close your eyes for a moment and visualise your inner cauldrons, one in your belly one at your heart and one at your head. Think about what feeds and nourishes these energy centres within you and what does not.

- ☾ What feeds your wellbeing – your cauldron of warming – and what drains it?

- ☾ What sparks joy in your heart, and what dampens it?

- ☾ What feeds your wisdom, and what pulls your attention away from what matters to you?

Take a piece of paper or your journal and draw the three cauldrons – either within a diagram of the body, or by themselves. Inside the cauldrons write or draw what fills them up. Outside the cauldrons write or draw the things that do not serve you. If you're not sure, or you find it distracting to categorise, you can simply use the space as one big cauldron.

After taking your time with this task, take a good look at what is outside your cauldrons and think of what you can let go of and may need to release. You may be in a job that drains your *qi* and does not nourish your true vocation. You may be so stressed and overworked that you feel exhausted and ungrounded. You may feel disconnected to your wisdom and crown chakra because you spend all day at a computer.

This exercise is not, by any means, an 'easy fix' but a tool to help you assess, explore and think about what changes you could make. This is all part of walking our path towards harmony. The more we can let fall by the wayside, the lighter we can travel in the direction we wish. It is common for people to get so dragged down in 'busy-ness' and ticking things off the to-do list that they have no time left even to decide where they really want to be headed, let alone check their path to get there.

Cauldron Questions (these may help with the activity above, or you can use them as journal prompts)

- What helps you feel safe and comforted? Money? Marriage? A support network of family? Carefully made plans?
- What nourishes you? Food, books, ideas, friends, sunshine…? Make a list.
- What stirs up your inner fire? What inspires you? What would you do every day if money was no object?
- What makes you feel connected to the universe? Do your thoughts support or criticise your dreams?

Be Your Own Lightworker

A Taoist master once gave this simple instruction:

Do not focus on being the healer – just be 'the Light'.

These magical cauldrons of energy can help us reflect on the idea of light as energy, and how we hold it within us. Where is your energy going? Is it being drained by holding onto grudges, fears and anxieties, or projects and connections that don't serve you? How can we lighten our load? How can we hold space and light for ourselves and others? How can we heal with this energy of lightness? What blocks can you clear out of the way to become a channel for that divine light of *shen* and personal power of *qi*?

Magic teaches us that things that seem to be impossible can become possible. Things that have become separated, blocked or broken, like people and energy, can be re-joined. We can find the light, find space and the empty cauldrons can be refilled with time and love. In the words of a well-known yogic mantra: "Live light, spread the light, be the light."

CLOSING YINSIGHTS

Through the day, and through our lives, we send out strands of energy in a million different ways – listening, travelling, creating, tending. Sometimes, we are sending out so much energy that we feel we have none left for ourselves.

If in doubt about how you are using your energy, a piece of advice that any witch would approve of, would be: 'come back to your cauldron'. These cauldrons are where we stir up our magic, where alchemy and transformation occur and where we can call our energy back home. Break strands if you need to, take time to refill and refuel. Tend to your own energy centres first, and then you can tend to others. Take your time and make your choices. When you decide to go out, embark on a big project, or go on an adventure you can go wholeheartedly, and fully with your awareness. Not half-heartedly and wishing you had stayed home with a book; this creates conflicts within us which is draining. And then when you do stay home with a book – do that wholeheartedly too! Try and let go of any guilt or fear that you are missing out!

6

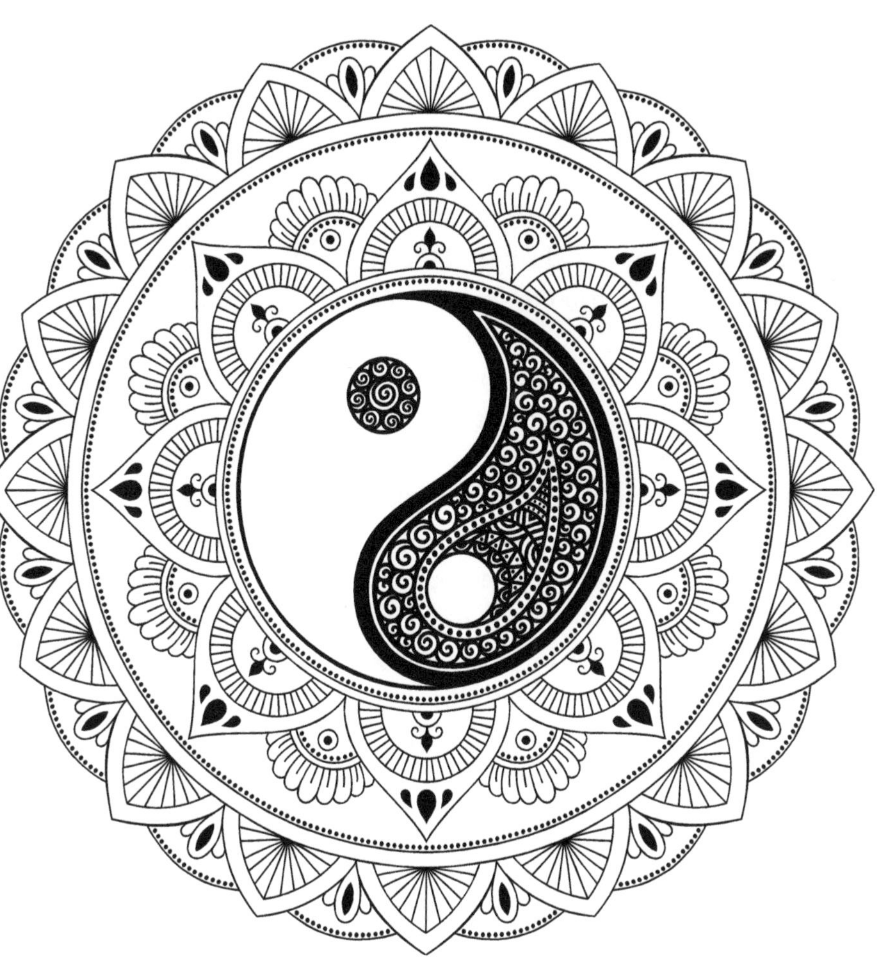

CULTIVATING THE PATIENCE OF NATURE

The valley spirit never dies;
It is the woman, primal Mother.
Her gateway is the root of heaven and earth.
It is like a veil barely seen.
Use it; it will never fail.
Tao Te Ching

You cannot force a flower to grow, all you can do is give it time. You cannot rush the seasons, they find their journey week by week. The cycles of moon, seasons and years can help us find more expansive schedules with which to synchronise, cycles a little more restful than the seconds, minutes, hours and workdays by which we currently order our days.

Whether we are waiting for bread to rise, seeds to germinate or plants to grow, we cannot force these things by willpower, or control – all there is to do is wait and listen to the pace of nature.

Yoga, Ayurveda, and Chinese medicine all work with the forces of nature. Working with nature occurs on both internal and external levels when it comes to balancing the energies of our own nature as body, mind, breath and spirit. Each of us is a manifestation of nature and living accordingly can help us in many ways.

Loving nature is one thing, learning from it is even better, and embracing a life lived in unity with the natural laws which govern the universe is the wisest action of all.

THE PACE OF *WU WEI*

Nature does not hurry
yet everything is accomplished.
Lao Tzu

The *Tao Te Ching* recommends learning non-action by observing the natural world. *Wu wei* shows that when we learn to wait and watch, we see outside forces more clearly and make wiser moves. Whereas when we act hastily, emotion and ego can drive our decisions. We, as humans, have a finite amount of energy (our *jing*: essence). With non-action, we conserve this precious energy so that we can utilise it at the right time; an essential skill of self-preservation.

It helps us to remember how to adapt ourselves to our environment and act according to the way nature encourages, rather than force it to our will, which is all too common in Western culture. Non-action goes against the Western ideal of working hard as the morally right thing to do; the grit and the hustle, pushing and striving. Tightening one's grip, trying to grasp and push is not the way to find harmony. Tao says we can let go of this effort, and allow ourselves to be carried, as though on a stream. *Wu wei* is a practice of acceptance of what is: an invitation to flow as nature unfolds. Letting go is not a weakness, laziness or passivity, but rather a wise form of strength to conserve one's energy.

We are all, at times, in danger of damaging ourselves through an overly unyielding adherence to ideas which cannot fit the demands of the world as it is, and ourselves, as we are. For instance, you may feel grief at the loss of a loved one or angry about an argument you had with a colleague. *Wu wei* suggests allowing yourself to accept these emotions as they come and go. Be present in the pain and anger that you are feeling. To try and resist them or ignore them creates a struggle like swimming against a current. Total bliss and harmony can't be found with *wu wei* alone – but this Taoist concept captures a pearl of distinctive wisdom we may at times be in great need of: to find calm as nature encourages us.

So how can we begin to practice this?

Listen to nature

You may find silence in nature… or beautiful sound: ocean waves, birdsong, leaves rustling, frogs and crickets singing. This can also help you connect with *your* stillness – see how the trees, while still, sway in a gentle breeze? Their stillness is different to the rocks, mountains and grass. Stillness is something you can feel within, and maybe you find it in different forms – what it looks like from outside, as always, matters not.

Try to find pockets of green

Wherever you live, find a green space to wander in, allowing yourself to drink in the beauty of the natural world. Connect to the yin elements of earth and water. Take your time to notice things that you may often overlook: the way the wind whips through branches; how frost catches the sunlight and sparkles; the joyful chatter of birds. The more you can stop thinking about your daily routine or work, and just savour the moment and what's in front of you, the more relaxed you can feel.

Water

If you can get into the sea or a lake, paddle in a babbling brook, walk beside a river or watch a fountain bubble, the idea of nature flowing gently is never clearer than through the beautiful yin element of water. In connecting to the qualities of water we can nurture them within ourselves: intuition, emotion and healing. In the Hindu tradition water is associated with Chandra, the moon deity who embodies spirit, transformation and yielding to change.

Light

Follow the circadian rhythms of the day. As it gets dark outside, see if you can do without much electric lighting and go instead for natural candlelight or fire if you are able. At the very least switch off the bright lights of iPhone, laptops and devices. This will help your body relax and prepare you for restful evening and sleep, as well as being a simple ritual to help you journey from the noise of the day into the restfulness of the night.

Wu wei with the seasons

Learning about living according to the seasons is *wu wei* in action, as well as a wonderful guide for our energy work through yoga, spellcraft and meditation.

One way of keeping yin and yang in harmonious balance is by studying and learning from nature how these two forces manifest and interact. We can observe that spring and summer represent yang (summer is the peak of yang), and late summer, autumn and winter represent yin (with winter being the peak of yin).

In observing both our inner natures and outer nature, we gain insight into certain emotions and reactions typical for a season, learning how to take care of ourselves and our inner life, by knowing each season.

The reward of living according to the seasons is nothing less than greater health and harmony.

The seasons transform into each other, as we saw in Chapter 2: winter (Water) gives birth to spring (Wood) and spring (Wood) gives birth to summer (Fire). The seasons shift and nature behaves in different ways with each season.

Spring means nature is turning green, and plants start to grow and expand. We should emerge into springtime having been restored by winter, ready to make plans and expand our energy. If we haven't rested enough during winter, we don't have that energy. And this is where it becomes a problem. If energy is depleted, it is not abundant for expansion and growth.

Then **summer** comes, and our energy should expand even further. Summer means spending time outdoors, living fully. It's warm, and nature is at peak yang energy. So should we be.

As summer comes to an end, a little season is noted in the Chinese year as **late summer**; known to some as Indian summer. This season begins in late August and goes through to autumn equinox. It belongs to the Earth element and is connected to harvest season. This fifth season provides amazing opportunities to nourish ourselves and express gratitude for the abundance we enjoy. Nature is starting to slow down and transition from yang to yin. We've gone through the Wood season during spring with a start of the yang energies – into fiery summer and the peak of yang – and now it's time to prepare ourselves for the beginning of the yin season with the Earth element.

During **autumn** we have the opportunity to let go of the things we no longer need, just as nature does. The trees don't hold on to their leaves, knowing that new leaves will bloom next season when spring arrives again. We humans could live accordingly: dropping whatever doesn't work for us. This is the time for introspection, meditation and ease.

Winter is the time for rest and rejuvenation. During winter, we may sleep more. Just looking at nature turning darker means we know it's rest season. What do many animals do during winter? They rest, many hibernating completely. Whereas we humans are expected to work as normal during winter. But there are still things we can do. Connect to the element of the season – Water. Go to sleep earlier. Eat soothing food. Spend more time at home. Go within. Meditate.

Modern life and societal pressures can keep us racing around. Always pushing and growing, whatever the time of year, like in the lead up to Christmas: we rush and plan and worry, until we burn out or get sick, and then get forced to rest and be still. This book is your invitation to live a little differently. To actively choose stillness and rest. To choose yin. So that when spring comes around once more, you will have the energy to start again.

SEASONAL CELEBRATION YIN SEQUENCES

You can tailor your yoga practice with the seasons in mind, celebrating the season you're in by tuning into its energy in your yoga practice.

By utilising yin yoga to work with seasonal energy, you can create more of the element/seasonal energy you desire. If you want to stimulate your creativity, you might want to connect with fiery summer energy. Or you may want to balance an element you feel you have too much of: if your thoughts are all over the place like springtime shoots and branches, you can carve away a little of the wood energy by working with the strength of autumn's metal energy.

SPRING/SUMMER SEQUENCE

This is the time of coming alive. To the witch, this is the season of the Goddess Brigid in her maiden aspect and Imbolc. After the yin of autumn-winter, the earth is filling with yang! This is a practice to allow you to rise with a connection to the earth, finding the yin way to rise.

In Chinese medicine, the months of spring and summer are related to the elements of Wood and Fire. According to the Celtic/Pagan Wheel of the Year, it's usually the elements of Air and Fire. All this wood, air and fire are what's needed for sparks to catch alight, to leave behind a little of the Water element of winter and ready for a new year to come to life!

The hip and front body openers here (Swan and Sphinx) connect to the energy flow of the Liver and Gallbladder meridians, the meridian of Wood representing germination, creation and growth. If you like to connect to ideas of the chakras, these poses also open the solar plexus and heart chakras.

Sphinx

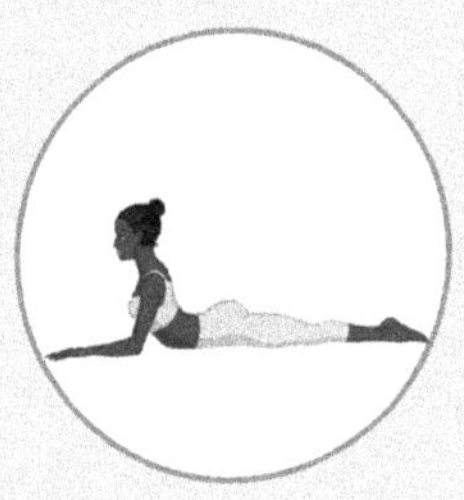

Opening through the heart and solar plexus. From lying on your stomach. Bring your forearms to the floor with your elbows under your shoulders, to raise your chest off the ground.

Garland Pose

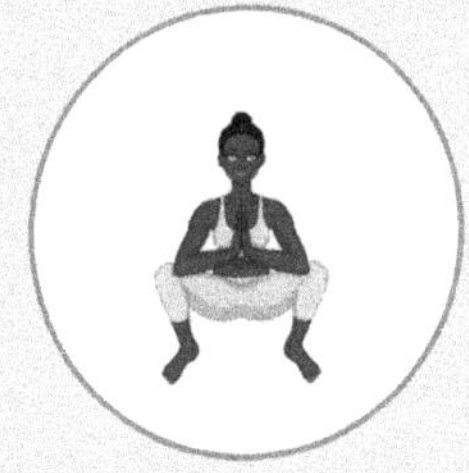

With feet a little wider than hips, we drop into a low squat, drawing the hands to prayer, long through the spine.

Cat and Cow

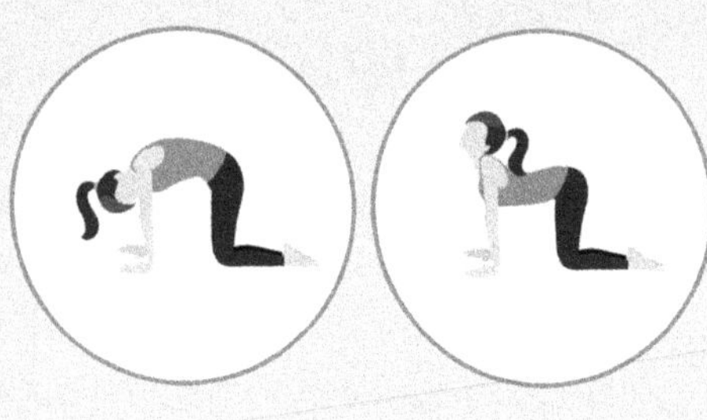

On all-fours, flex the spine inward and outwards with the breath. A little dynamic movement, just to bring in a tiny bit of yang!

Toe Stretch

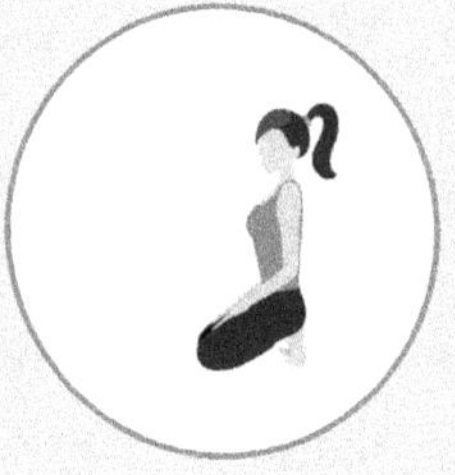

Stretching through the soles of the feet, activating the meridian lines for the Liver, Spleen and Kidneys. Tuck the toes under and then sit back on the heels with the spine tall.

Swan and Sleeping Swan

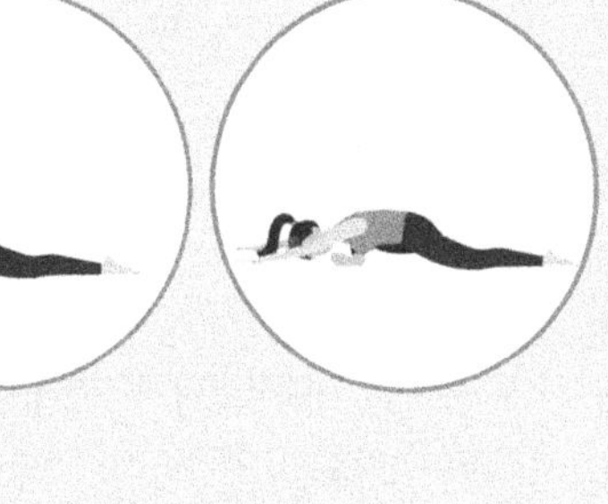

As correspondence to Goddess Brigid, the Swan is a gorgeous pose to bring into spring and summer yin practice. As a symbol, the swan represents beauty, love, and strength.

From hands and knees, slide your right knee behind your right wrist. And bring the right foot forward, towards the left wrist, aiming to keep the hips square. Slide the left knee away to open hips towards the earth.

From here you can stay supported on hands or melt the body down onto forearms or rest on the earth (known as Sleeping Swan).

AUTUMN/WINTER SEQUENCE

On the Celtic/Pagan Wheel of the Year, autumn and winter relate to elements of Water and Earth. In Chinese medicine, they are Metal and Water. Water, in both cultures, represents transformation, healing and yielding. Earth is groundedness and Metal can be a carrier for water and a symbol of strength. These elements share the corresponding chakras: the Root (Earth) and Sacral (Water) chakras.

Hip and thigh openers like Dragon and Dragonfly can connect to the Stomach and Spleen meridians and can help soothe worry and anxiety. This always makes me think of 'rest and digest' (when the Sympathetic Nervous System is activated, and the body is relaxed and functioning optimally) the opposite of 'fight or flight' stress response. In releasing the tension of the hips, we may find our way to a calmer place: to digest our food, but also digest what we have drawn in and learnt over the active months of spring and summer.

Dragonfly

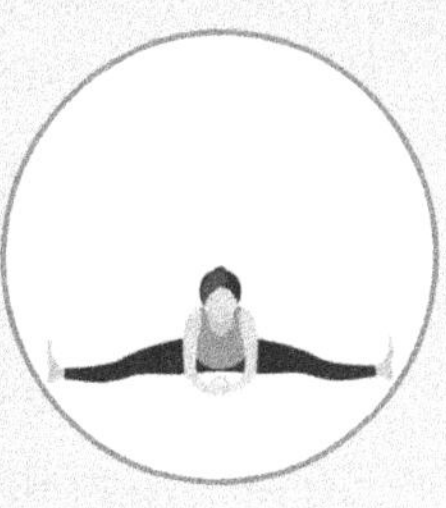

Wide-legged fold. From seated take your legs as wide as is comfortable. Keeping your legs straight and toes pointing towards the sky, hinging from the hips walk your hands forward to a comfortable fold, let the neck be soft and your head fall forward.

Shoelace

From seated, bend your knees and put your soles on the earth. Bring your left foot under the right knee to the outer right hip. Cross your right leg over the left, stacking the right knee on top of the left, the right foot comes to the outside of the left hip. Sit evenly on the sitting bones. Work with sitting in this way for a minute or more.

Lizard

This low-to-the-earth lunge invites us to open through the hips. Start on your hands and knees. Step your left foot to the ground outside your left hand. Bring this foot forward until the knee is above the ankle. Slide the right knee backward as far as you can. You may keep your hands on the ground or on blocks. Or bring your elbows to the earth. Bring in the support of a blanket or cushion under the back knee if needed.

Caterpillar/Forward Fold

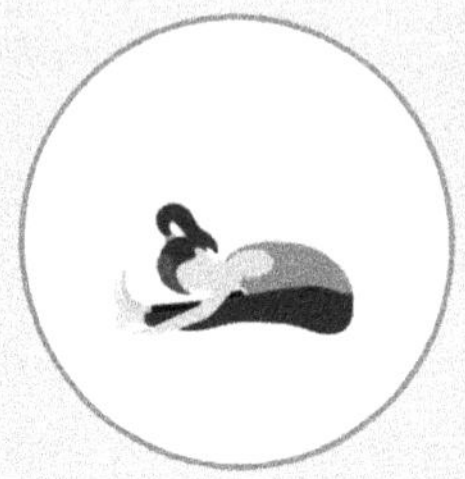

From seated, extend your legs out in front of you, hinging from the hips into a forward fold, letting the head hang heavy.

Reclining Butterfly

Also known as Reclining Goddess. Lying on your back, bring the soles of the feet together and your hands resting above your head to make two mirroring diamonds. You can also let your hands fall to your sides or use support as shown here if that feels more restful.

WHEEL OF THE YEAR

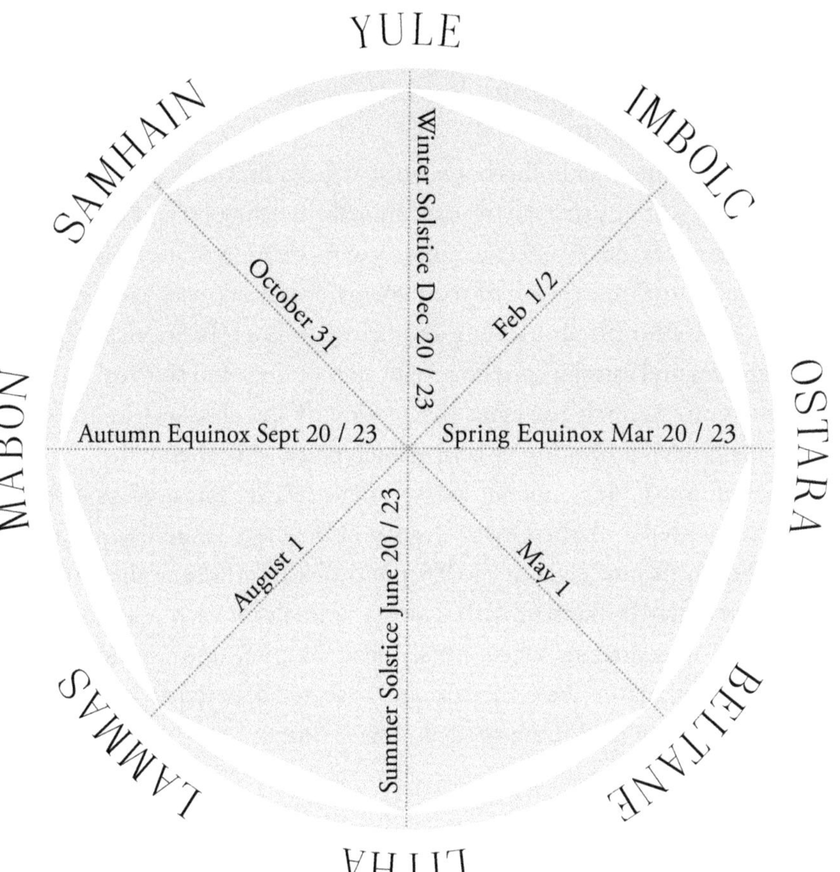

(for the southern hemisphere version see sentiayoga.com/yinmagic)

ANIMAL NATURE

You will notice that many of the postures in yin yoga take their names from animals. When we practice them, we can allow ourselves to be aware of and connect to the distinctive physical and energetic qualities of these animals.

All of the practices in this book: yoga, witchcraft, Celtic and Chinese cultural traditions strongly feature animals in symbolic and energetic ways. Witches may connect to animals in meditation or use feathers or bones in ritual to connect to their energy or powers, such as strength or vision. Animals also feature in ancient texts of Taoist alchemists, magicians and astrologers who sought immortality and spiritual transformation. Animals represent the motion of the elements in action, each animal representing its own elemental *wu xing* energy.

In ancient China, animals are, among other things, used as directional symbols – Azure/Green Dragon of the East, Vermillion Bird of the South, White Tiger of the West and Black Tortoise of the North. And you may be familiar with Chinese animals for each year: rat, ox, tiger, rabbit, dragon, snake, horse, goat, monkey, rooster, dog, pig. Like star signs in Western culture, these are believed to symbolise personality traits of those born at certain times.

THE NATURAL BODY

Whilst seeking animals as teachers can remind us of a more primal, instinctive way of being, it is important to remember that it is our own natures we must get in touch with, rather than simply pretending to be other animals or idealising nature outside of ourselves. We are indivisible from nature, we just forget this!

In Hindu philosophy it is said that we are made up of three components: the energy body, the physical body and *karana sarira* – the natural body. From Sanskrit, *karana* translates as "causing" or "making" – our natural body is connected to our intrinsic nature. *Karana sarira* is considered the seed from which our energy and physical

Tiger and Dragon

The *I Ching* uses animal imagery – the dragon and tiger – to portray the yin-yang dynamic. They represent the interplay that is observed through the natural world. These are the two pathways of power: the yin way and the yang way, tiger way and dragon way.[i]

Tiger

The tiger carries yin energy, embodying the qualities of courage, purpose and patience – much as a tiger deliberately and patiently stalks its prey. Its power is coiled and hidden deep within, but a tiger can spring into action at will. Along with being a yin animal, the tiger also represents the direction of the west and feminine energy. Tiger is an Earth creature and more grounded than the dragon, she is also connected to the yin element of Metal.

Dragon

The dragon is a creature of yang, symbolic of masculine, sky/heaven centred energy, bravery and good fortune. The dragon is powerful, adventurous and outgoing. The dragon's corresponding direction is east, place of the rising sun, directly opposite to the tiger. One may connect the dragon to yang elements of Fire and Wood as the dragon can be fiery and destructive.

....

i Note: these pairings are drawn from the *I Ching* text that connects dragon with Heaven and the masculine, and Tiger with Earth and feminine. But I have seen these animals swapped round and differing in their representations in other texts – dragon as yin, slow and steady in its lumbering walk, resting in pools and only breathing fire when absolutely necessary and connected to earth element and the leaping tiger as yang and the wood element. So as always, your interpretation/cultural sources may differ from what I am sharing here.

body grow. It contains the *samskara* and *karma* – impressions of experience and actions, including through our ancestors and bloodlines. *Karana sarira* may be considered a gateway, a connection to the patterns and rhythms of our lives through time.

You'll note the word "seed" is used to describe our natural body, a word also commonly used to describe the Chinese concept of *jing*; both use the patterns of nature to define our energy and where its drawn from. This is an important reminder to us that the possibilities and seeds of potential are held within each of us. Seeds have within them not only this *potential* for growth but also the memory, the *instinct* of how to grow, how to move towards the light.

It can be a challenge to connect to our roots, to the seeds of our being, and the roots that run into our history and generations before us. We have been taught in so many ways to avoid this. But as we practice, we begin to connect more deeply with who we are and what matters most to us, allowing us to discard things that don't matter and focus our energy in a way that is in harmony with our nature, as part of the natural world. In doing so we stop the most essential of battles, which humans seem unique in: fighting the expression of our innate selves.

In the natural world, it can be scary facing a shifting ocean or vast mountain or lashing rain, and it can be the same when facing parts of yourself; your shifting anger, vast power, lashing grief, but they are not 'bad', they are to be respected, but not feared. They are simply elements of nature and your energy, your journey, your experiences. To embrace emotion, (rather than deny or dissociate) is to truly connect and activate our spiritual and natural power. With stillness and strength, we can face that 'mountain' whether it be a mountain of emotion or a mountain of rock and earth.

The Disconnect

More and more we may find ourselves, whether intentionally or not, cut off from the natural rhythms and cycles of nature and our bodies. We no longer get up with the sun, instead we stay up till the small hours of the morning with our phones lighting up our faces, or trying to finish one final spreadsheet for work. Our bodies may well be disconnected from daily rhythms, no longer recognising whether it is day or night. This happens when we expose ourselves to bright lights and vigorous exercise at night and then feel unable to sleep, because the body is disconnected from the natural process of slowing down and dimming light that happens as night rolls in.

With this disconnect, lunar phases may go unnoticed, new seasons unacknowledged. This can disrupt our body clocks, creating stressful lives in discord with the natural rhythms that govern all life. Like two different drumbeats fighting to create a tune. Disconnection to many, has become normal.

Once, all cultures would have lived guided by the natural cycles, using celebrations, festivals, and outdoor ritual to mark the changing of rhythms through the year. Most of these are now lost to our current striving lives. We can bring these traditions back by marking them with simple, joyful activities. For example, celebrating the solstices and equinoxes by holding a ritual supper, a gathering of friends or ceremony of gratitude, or a simply a walk to watch the sunrise on these special days.

CLOSING YINSIGHTS

If we do not utilise natural prompts and invitations to rest, we may be unable to use strength and action when we need it. For example, if, instead of sleeping we spend half the night scrolling through the internet or replaying an argument in our minds, we will not feel rested to take on the challenges of the next day.

So, take time to connect to the energy and transitions of each of the seasons, they are invaluable in teaching and guiding us. We can utilise our yin yoga practice to mirror the seasonal energy around us. If in doubt look to nature, because, and this is always good to remember, *we are nature!* Spend more time in your garden or a local park, or start a window box to allow plants to guide you through, seeing the seasons within their leaves and flowers. To connect to the rhythm of nature is to connect to life. We are not separate, although we can feel separated. Connect to nature within and outside of yourself – we are all connected.

7

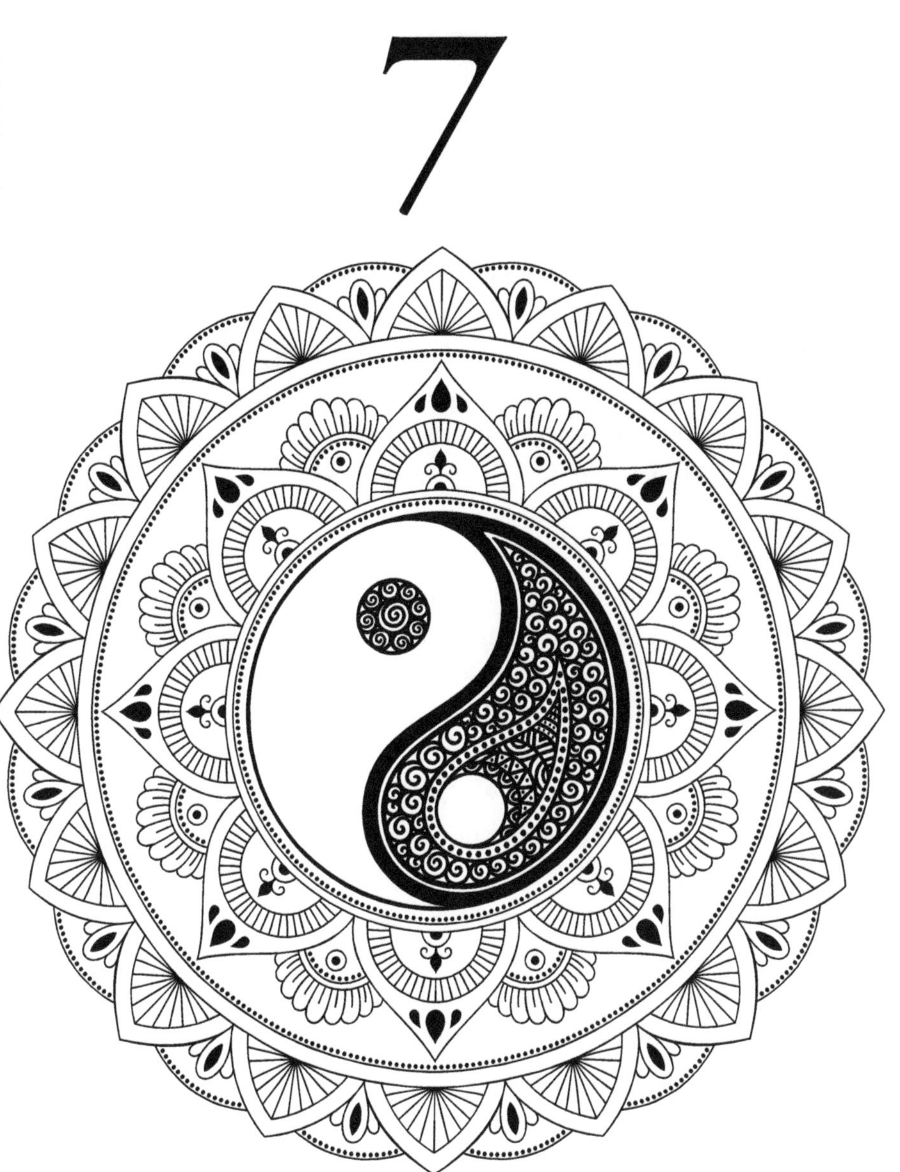

SYMPATHETIC MAGIC

Sympathetic magic is a type of magic based on imitation or connection. It appears in similar forms throughout all cultures and eras: it seems almost innate to us as humans. The term "sympathy" means to enter into another being's mental state and feel affinity and compassion for their being. So, with yin yoga, you are practicing a simple and beautiful form of sympathetic magic, because the being you are connecting to and showing compassion for is yourself and your existence. This is something that we don't do often enough!

Sympathetic magic is also the belief that a person or object can be affected magically by actions performed towards something that represents them, such as work with dolls or poppets that represent real people (usually not for malicious purposes, despite how they are often portrayed).

The earliest forms of sympathetic magic may well be ancient treasures such as prehistoric cave drawings and carvings of the goddess. Archaeologists believe that many ancient cave paintings are the result of seeking successful hunts; the shaman or tribe elder would perform a ritual before a pursuit in which a bountiful trip is acted out and create images of the hunters successfully killing their prey. And icons of the goddess may have been a way to seek her favour or blessing, offerings to the icon representing offerings to the goddess herself.

Sympathetic magic has existed for millennia, but its name may have been first articulated in the modern Western tradition in a book called *The Golden Bough* (1890) which featured two fundamental principles which we now call the Law of Similarity and the Law of Contact.

The Law of Similarity states very simply that 'like produces like'. We can use these ideas in magic if we wish to effect a change: creating our intention through symbolic action. An example might be a witch who wants to buy her 'dream house'. She may paint an image of the house with herself standing joyfully in the doorway, holding a bunch of flowers grown from its garden. Or maybe more relevant to our yin journey, you can create a ritual of cultivating self-love. Even when you may not necessarily feel that love, you are creating that intention and cultivating it through symbolic action, as something to work towards. Positive affirmations and visualisations could also be called sympathetic magic as we seek to produce an effect we desire by imitating it in our mind's eye.

Another aspect of the Law of Similarity is that things that are connected can bring about similar effects. This idea is also the basis of correspondences. For example, the element of fire can be represented by a collection of items that represent the energy of the fire element such as sun images, incense, fire opal and fiery spices. They all have the power to 'ignite' the body and psyche as fire does.

Sympathetic magic comes naturally to us if we let it. We instinctively know how to create groups and patterns from things found in the natural world through association of colour, form or qualities. For example, many of us could easily come up with ten items connected to the sun via association (like sunflowers, animals, fruits, seeds, colours, candles, seasons, zodiac signs) with little or no prior magical knowledge. These would be just the kind of resources used in sympathetic magic.

The second principle of sympathetic magic is the Law of Contact. This is the understanding that things that have been in contact with each other continue to share a connection of energy. Therefore, what is done to an object could affect the person/object with which it once had contact. When performing a spell, the practitioner may have something personal such as a lock of hair, clothing, photograph, for whom the spell is being cast. A yogi may treasure a mala necklace gifted to them by their guru or teacher, and feel in some way the knowledge and inspiration of their teacher is with them when they have their necklace near.

SYMPATHETIC MAGIC FOR YOGA

Create a symbolic totem for your yin yoga practice using the laws of similarity. This can be done by creating your own mala necklace to wear or have near you in your yoga practice. Mala bead necklaces are traditionally made with 108 *rudraksha* seeds which symbolise clarity and calm, as well as a connection to the Hindu god Shiva. The myth tells that from deep meditation, Lord Shiva opened his eyes and a teardrop fell to the earth. The teardrop formed the seeds that became the *rudraksha* tree. So, in a form of sympathetic magic used by ancient yogis, the *rudraksha* bead malas would help form a similarity or connection between the wearer and the qualities of the god Shiva, supporting the yogi's journey of meditation.

You can make your mala necklace using any beads that are in some way associated with what you wish to connect to. Here are some examples that align with our yin-seeking purposes:

- Cedarwood beads: connected to grounding, stability and also awareness. Great for seeking insight or truth.
- Lava stone beads: lava stone is a natural black rock formed from volcanic magma. It results in beads that have irregular surfaces, making each one unique. Lava stone is grounding, connected to the root chakra in this combination of fire and earth.
- Jade: connected to wisdom, healing, courage, love and long life.
- Pearls: connected to the element of water, for wisdom, healing, transformation and clarity of mind.
- Black onyx: a powerful healing and grounding stone. In the Chinese tradition it is considered yin and is associated with protection and grounding.

Feel free to use only as many beads as you wish. This doesn't have to cost much. You could repurpose beads from an old necklace, or even just have one little bead on a chain to keep in your pocket!

When creating your necklace, think about imbuing the process with your intentions. What are you seeking? Greater balance? Less guilt about taking time for yourself? Healing rest?

THE SYMPATHETIC MAGIC OF THE NERVOUS SYSTEM

Our nervous systems – the aptly named sympathetic and parasympathetic systems, that we explored together in Chapter 1 – work in sympathy with our reactions and emotions: they are their own kind of sympathetic magic.

'Sympathy' like the word yoga, means connection. We often think of sympathy as being an emotional connection to someone, but it can also be an energetic or spiritual connection. In the context of this practice, that 'someone' is you! So, in our yoga here in these pages and beyond, we are seeking sympathy and connection with our body: listening, hearing and loving our body.

On our yoga mat, we can connect to the nervous system and sympathetic magic. The Law of Contact reminds us that we can imbue the space where we practice and our yoga mat with calm and clarity, and every time we come back there, we can pick up a little of that energy. The Law of Similarity tells us that we can connect to, and embody, the groundedness of earth, connecting to the surety of the earth in our practice. We can use our practice as a symbolic action, practising treating ourselves with patience and forgiveness, even when we don't always feel that way.

The following are other simple, great ways to activate the parasympathetic nervous system, enabling us to rest and digest:

Sitting with Emotion

Being still often means emotions come up that we may have keeping ourselves busy to avoid – but that the body and mind need to process. I think this is one of many reasons people find slow, meditative yoga practice so challenging. To sit with sorrow, anger or guilt is not always that appealing, as vital as it may be.

There is, however, value in what we may call our 'negative emotions' and to thrive and live a life of meaning requires embracing the darkness (I'll talk more about this in Chapters 8 and 9), not exclusively seeking out the light. Sitting with emotion can teach us to see the value in negative emotions rather than always seeking to avoid them. Anger can be energising and empower you to take action against injustice, and guilt can prompt you to seek forgiveness, grow and change. If we spend our lives avoiding emotions like disappointment and self-doubt, we might never take on new challenges, depriving ourselves of the chance to develop in new ways. Embracing these feelings is not about being 'tough' or 'strong', but creating space for emotions to happen and unfurl. We can create suffering for ourselves by wishing things were different, by blaming others, by fighting what's happening – especially when we so often seek that 'ideal life' that society and the media would have us believe exists. Challenging emotions cannot be 'solved', they must be felt, journeyed through and, in your own time, healed. It is a journey, and you will arrive at your destination different from where you started. So when you experience challenges, pain, sorrow, please treat yourself with kindness and self-compassion, take your time to feel and be still, to experience, learn and grow.

Daydream

Within the brain, neurons in their billions interact through synaptic connections. These neurons, like all things in nature, grow, adapt and also die – with each new experience and memory, the brain rewires its physical structure. So, the more we think, imagine and reflect, the stronger and more complex our neural networks become.

There are specific central regions of the brain that help us imagine the thoughts and feelings of others, draw on memory and experience. These areas combined are known as our 'default mode network', and this is where the brain's energy goes to when focused consciousness switches off: it is sort of the opposite of mindfulness, as we have no focused attention. We wouldn't want to move through our day in this state, but time to let the mind wander can be useful: it allows thoughts, ideas and images to flow through our mind's eye. As we let the mind wander, truths and intuition can be revealed. Slipping into trance-like states can help us to seek messages from other realms or times, a skill practiced by oracles, hedge witches, shamans and mediums the world over.

Here we can connect once more to sympathetic magic as we may connect to the energies of others, or cultivate manifestations using positive visualisation. Through day dream, we can wander through time, plan our futures based on past experiences, reflect on mistakes we have made, inhabit the minds of others, increasing empathy and understanding, allowing us to create new ideas, stories and possibilities.

Just Breathe...

Changes in breathing, what yogis know as *pranayama* – breathing at different paces or paying careful attention to the breath – engage different parts of the brain. Humans' ability to consciously control and regulate their breathing is unique and can have a profound effect on our feelings and behaviour. Even merely focusing on one's breathing allows synchrony between brain areas and improved brain function: greater focus, calmness, and emotional control. Brain scans of breathwork offer scientific confirmation of what meditators and yogis already know: during times of stress, or when focus is needed, mindfulness on one's breathing allows greater access to the full abilities of our mind and the mind-body connection.

Taoist Meditation

If you want more structured meditation ideas, Taoism contains many meditation techniques, including concentration, mindfulness, contemplation and visualisation.

Taoist meditation practices begin with the following three premises:

1. The mind must focus on something.
2. The body must become relaxed.

3. The breath must become slow, soft and even.

Mind, body, breath need to be regulated until harmony is reached. In this process, as the mind instructs the body to relax, the breathing will slow. If the breathing slows, the body relaxes. When the body is calm, the mind can focus more efficiently. Once the first three states are 'achieved', two more states can be cultivated:

4. Regulating *qi*.

5. Regulating *shen*.

As we breathe in, we draw in *qi*. This flows into the lungs, starting the process of storing of *qi* into the cauldron of the *xia tan tien* (which we explored in Chapter 5) so that it can circulate through the body and mind and onto greater awareness of consciousness.

Other types of meditation

- **Emptiness meditation** – This meditation is about learning stillness, calming the body and letting go of all thoughts and feelings to find inner quiet and emptiness. This state allows for spiritual energy to be refreshed and replenished.
- **Breathing meditation** – Many traditions, including Hinduism, use this technique. Focusing on the breath, uniting it with *qi*/*prana*. Like the Buddhist practice *samatha*, which can be translated as "concentration", where controlled focus is brought to one thing – a chant, a candle flame, the breath, and letting go of all other thoughts and perceptions.
- **Inner vision** – A process of seeing our true path/dharma/Tao using our mind's eye to travel through the wilds of our emotions and inner being. Using the mind's eye is also used in yoga nidra and guided meditation journeys.
- **Insight Meditation** – known as *vipassana* to yogis and Buddhists. Bringing awareness of exactly what is happening as it happens. This is not about emptying the mind but noticing all sensations, the comings and goings of the mind, how your body

feels and the sensations of the world around you.

Yogic Insight to Meditation

Pratyahara

These Taoist approaches – especially emptiness meditation – are ways to journey to what a yogi would call *pratyahara* or the 'withdrawal of the senses'. *Pratyahara* is the fifth 'limb' of the eight branches of Patanjali's outline of yoga (as mentioned in his foundational text, *The Yoga Sutras*). It's a little like a hermit crab withdrawing into its shell – limbs and senses all draw inwards until your whole world becomes this space within.

Our society operates by exciting our interest through the senses. We are faced with constant stimulation: bright colours, loud noises, information, pictures of perfect lives and shocking headlines. All of us at some point in our lives, (and many of us pretty regularly) experience sensory overload: the result of constant stimulus of our senses from TV, computers, adverts and social media.

So it's no wonder that drawing the senses away from all this 'noise' is a challenge. Have you heard the phrase "it's like herding cats"? That's what it's like trying to herd the senses inwards! Every time you manage to get one going in the right direction, other ones leap out of your arms, or knock the TV remote off of a table, or chase a splash of light on the floor... you get the idea!

The difficulty is that the senses have their own will, chiefly instinctual in nature. And if we don't actively work towards controlling them, they dominate and distract us with their endless demands (this also sounds a lot like cats!) And many of us who struggle with finding stillness within are so accustomed to ongoing sensory activity that we don't really know how to keep our minds quiet. In constantly attending to the senses we tend to forget our higher purpose or dharma.

For our journey to find stillness *pratyahara* is a vital limb of yoga. And the practice of *pratyahara* via meditation can help us work towards releasing environmental and sensory 'noise' and opening up to our inner being.

Sakshi

Sakshi is a yogic term for being a witness, a watcher, observing from an objective place, which admittedly, is not easy! Like *pratyahara*, it's about taking a step back. To observe instead of constantly being in reaction to our surroundings (which can be exhausting). Viewing our situation from a distance allows us to witness a situation in its entirety, expanding our perspective and insight. Maybe this helps us to see things a little more clearly. And possibly within this observation, we may discover or remind ourselves that there is no 'perfect', and there is no objective measure of 'right'. The natural world, society and the human condition present us with opportunities; from here relationships with others and ourselves consist of the choices we make.

It's possible that in meditation practices such as this, you may discover how much your mind distorts the reality you perceive. We can project our own subjective thoughts onto a reality we have created in our own minds. What we see, hear and feel is not really objective: but often coloured with, fears, anxieties and shadows we hold without even realizing. This is another vital way to explore finding our peace with things.

Vipassana meditation is closely linked with *sakshi*: it is also known as Insight Meditation; as a practice of clearing of the mind to seek insight into one's true nature and the true nature of reality. *Vipassana*, like *sakshi*, is both a process and a destination: to see things as they truly are.

In yoga and Hindu spiritual practice, the yogi seeks to become an unbiased observer of their thoughts, breath and body; to rest in pure awareness. When you are aware and no longer caught up in the noise of the world, you may ask yourself such questions as: *Is this an emotion I need to feel? Do I need to journey with it? Or is it something I can release?*

YIN SOUL AND THE MOTHERLINE

As part of this sympathy towards ourselves and to those around us in our practice of sympathetic magic, we cannot leave out our ancestors and our connection to them, both via thought and energy. Ancestors, as in many cultures, have a huge importance in Taoist theology. Not least in reference to the soul, which has within it; yin and yang components: *hun* – the yang, dynamic, 'cloud-soul' and *po* – the yin, the grounded, physical/bodily 'white-soul'.

Hun is home to our karma, so that's the part of the soul that reincarnates into new physical bodies, with a new consciousness. The *po* part of your soul remains in the earth and spirit realm. This suggests that it is the yin part of the soul that remembers who you are, where and who you came from.

This yin element of the soul joins the ancestral energy and memory of the universe, which, to my mind, is like the motherline and matriarchal lineage of women and witches alike.

We often think of ourselves as individuals, but our life force has passed down the generations to get to us. Some of our power and magic have journeyed through generations to arrive here. Our bodies and minds hold the memories of many generations that have gone before us, which is empowering and exciting. But other things, such as trauma also pass down the generations, which may be daunting (but certainly not insurmountable) as we seek to heal.

The idea of the motherline is backed up by science. In reproduction, the mitochondria, which cells use as a source of energy, are inherited exclusively from the mother (this is true for humans and many other mammals as well). These mitochondria continue to work for us our entire lives, drawing energy from our food for us to use. That's right, they are little energy centres you could envisage as teeny tiny cauldrons! The fact that mitochondria are maternally inherited enables genealogists to trace maternal lineage back through females. They have been used to track the ancestry of many species back hundreds of generations.

You possess a maternal inheritance, whether you are aware of it or not. A maternal line exists within you – both on a cellular and energetic level. We can harness this motherline energy through a spell of sympathetic magic. You may light a candle for your foremothers whenever you wish, to feel a connection, and to nurture healing, and to reconnect to where and how you have been held.

When I was training to be a Priestess of Brigid, we each had to create our own motherline ceremony, making representations of every woman in our motherline and petitioning for healing for them all. I share with you the prayer that I wrote for it.

I light this candle for every mother and woman in my motherline, lost and found, risen up and come to ground. The feeders and the fighters. Those that try so hard. Thank you, mothers. I love you all.

This is obviously very personal to me, but when writing this section, I felt I couldn't leave it out, and it may be of use to you too if you would like to create your own ceremony.

Motherline in Yoga

An awareness of our maternal heritage adds a whole other perspective on things we may be releasing, working through, listening to during our yoga practice, reminding us why we need to be kind and patient with ourselves. The tension, pain and trauma we are releasing may be generations old. It's also a reminder if you feel emotions coming up and you have no idea where they are coming from. You may be releasing something long held, not just by you – it's wonderful, and healing, but it can be confusing, and even overwhelming. So, use kindness and patience, let it flow, whatever comes up. You can stop your practice and come back to it tomorrow – little by little, step by step. But we need that stillness to connect and hear this memory of the motherline and our own specific lineage of feminine wisdom.

As we seek connection through magic and yoga work, we are always in the presence of, not just in our immediate surroundings, but with our links to our past, the flow of energy through generations. Via yoga and magical practice we can connect to our roots, ancestors and the earth. We are reconnecting to the story of our origin, drawing together into wholeness and the peace inherent in that.

MOTHERLINE YIN YOGA SEQUENCE

This reflection on the motherline inspired me to create a yin yoga sequence, so we can move and embody this flow of the motherline through the cycles of life and embrace the energy of nurturing. In this sequence we journey in a cycle from *savasana* (also known quite powerfully as Corpse Pose) to a rebirth in the Fetal and Happy Baby Poses, to Child's Pose, Goddess Pose and back to *savasana*. This sequence shows how you can utilise the ideas of yin yoga and, as I have, bring in ideas of sacred cycles of the divine feminine.

Try to settle into each pose for 3 minutes or more, take your time to find your connections.

Savasana/pose of relaxation

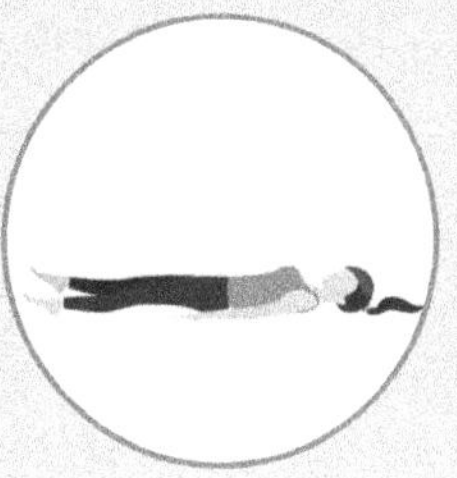

Lying on the ground connect to earth and the ancestors, letting all you do not need to fall away.

Fetal Pose

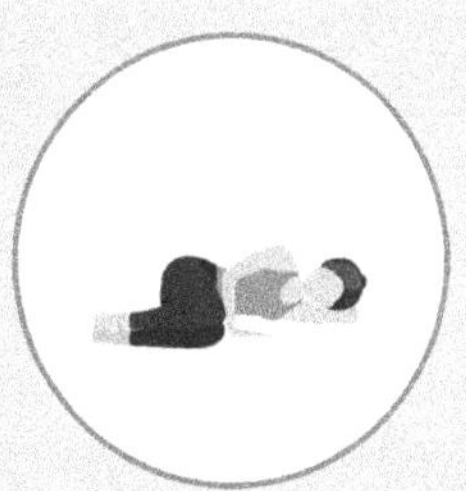

From *savasana* bend your knees, so the soles of the feet are on the floor. Roll to one side. From *savasana* we are being reborn. You can bring a pillow under your head for support. Be sure to spend time on both sides.

Happy Baby

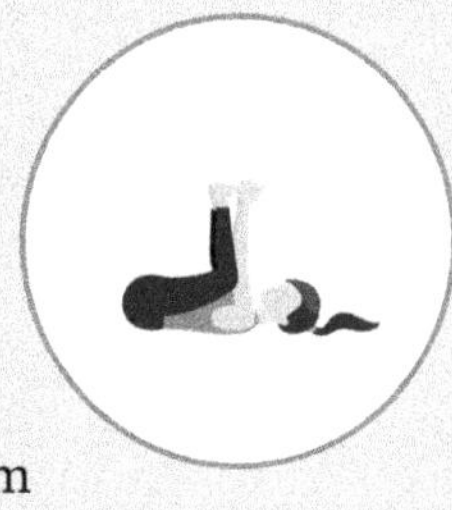

Roll onto your back. Draw your knees in towards your armpits, opening through the hips. Shining the soles of the feet to the sky, hold the outer edges of the feet. If this feels too much, you can do Half Happy Baby, holding onto the knees, drawing them in toward your armpits.

Child's Pose

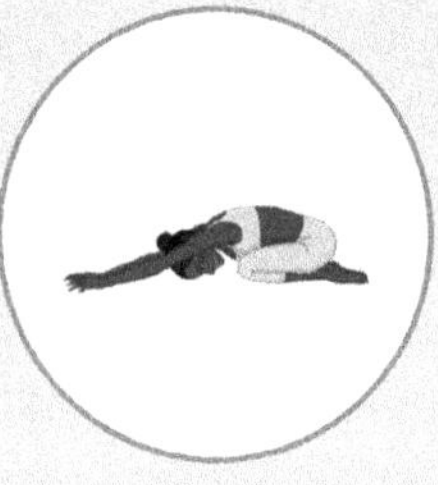

Make your way up to all fours and then drop your bum back onto your heels. With your arms you can either reach the hands forward or towards the toes, both are lovely versions of the pose.

Seated Goddess

Usually known as the Butterfly in yin yoga, but her goddess name is my personal favourite and seemed most appropriate here.

From seated, put the soles of your feet together, drawing your heels towards your hips and opening your knees towards the earth. Rise tall through your spine, let your shining crown rise to the sky. You are goddess, woman, queen.

Savasana/pose of relaxation

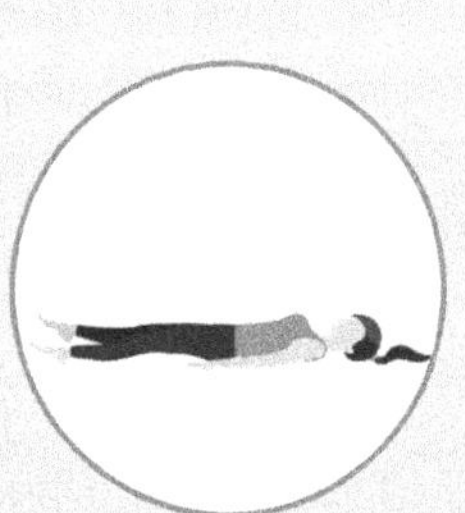

We come full cycle and return to the earth, resting.

CLOSING YINSIGHTS

Sympathetic magic is very simply about connection – connection between things and between people – helping us feel as they feel, connecting to their energy. And as we as yogis seek most often – connection to and of elements of our own energy.

Connection to ourselves is powerful, for in connecting to ourselves we connect to our ancestors, for we are all of them. For women, the motherline is the living knowledge of ourselves as alchemical cauldrons and potential carriers of life. Every woman is connected to the women before her through the roots, magic and flow of energy through generations, skills, ideas and memories passed down through bloodlines. A magical amount of power and connection lays within our ancestral bonds – like witchcraft itself, the knowledge can travel through us in many ways.

The soul remembers, and whether you feel within yourself one soul, two or many more, you can unite with all souls from your ancestral cauldron, for healing, release, connection and comfort. Many of us may have histories that we do not or cannot know much about, but you still connect intuitively, on a soul level. Much, and maybe all, of what we truly need to know is already within us.

8

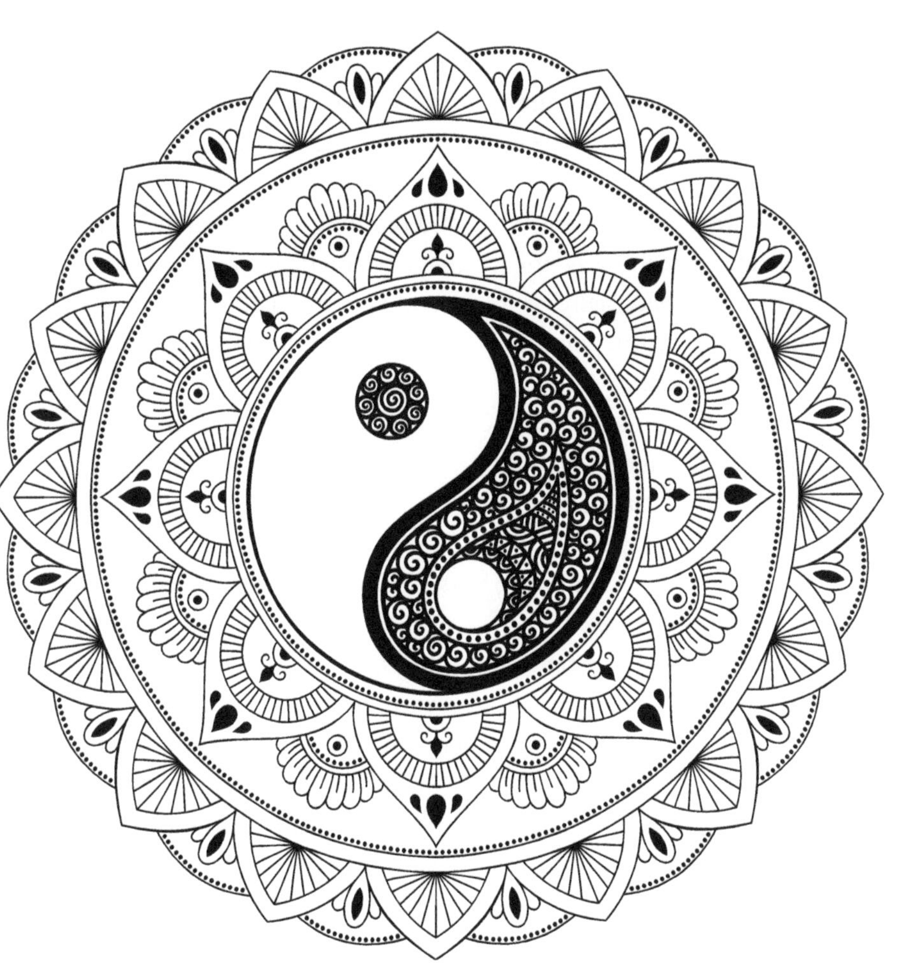

DARK MAGIC

Night is when we are closer to ourselves, closer to essential ideas and feelings that do not register so much during daylight hours.

Clarissa Pinkola Estes, *Women Who Run with the Wolves*

So far in this book, my darlings, we have explored the history and philosophy of the word yin. And the magical world of Taoism that it is drawn from. We have explored together how teachers have taken the essence of this word and created beautiful things like yin yoga.

Now we've taken in the 'what' and the 'why' of yin and its benefits, how can we really get into revelling, celebrating, luxuriating in the innate yin-ness of daily, monthly and yearly cycles? How might the witch embrace this yin world and take advantage of yin times for their own benefit?

The name of this chapter does not, as you may have guessed, refer to the use of dark magic for destruction or harm. I do not support magic for revenge or cruelty, however much we believe it is deserved. This is about the magic *of* the dark, and made *with* the dark. For me, the real magic of the dark is in facing fears, shadows and stillness and finding power within them.

Yin has qualities of darkness, stillness, of the hidden and the quiet. Dark times: the new moon, winter, night-time – are all times traditionally associated with witchcraft and women's magic – that can naturally help us connect to our yin, at a yin time.

Within this chapter we will explore the yin times of night, new moon and winter. These three yin stages are obviously varied in their regularity. Within each 24-hour day, you'll enjoy some night time (except residents of Northern Scandinavia and the Arctic Circle at certain times of the year!). Every lunar month you'll get to experience the new moon. And every year – unless you live on the equator[i] – you

i If you don't experience winter where you live, you can work with hours of the day. Between 5 and 7pm is connected to the Water element in Chinese elemental theory (each day journeys though all of the *Wu Xing* elements in cycle).

will have wintertime. Understanding yin can be a helping hand on the journey of experiencing stillness and making magic, or a chance to appreciate these times in a new way.

There is such value in understanding and connecting to the cycles and seasons of the year. No one can 'hold back the tide'. Our lives can be a discovery, a dance and harmonising rhythm with these natural cycles, or it can be a constant battle. As always, it's up to us. Just as with our yin and yang, this is not a battle between two elements but a journey to find a perfect point of balance between them. This is a possibility for moving in cycles of serenity and acceptance.

Meeting the Shadow Self

Filling the conscious mind with ideal conceptions is a characteristic of Western theosophy, but not the confrontation with the shadow and the world of darkness. One does not become enlightened by imagining figures of light, but by making the darkness conscious.

Carl Jung

I mentioned in Chapter 5 about Carl Jung and his insightful ideas about alchemy as a tool for inner transformation work. He was also the pioneer of an idea that is commonly used within magical work and Western psychology: the 'shadow self', using the term 'the shadow' to describe those aspects of our personalities that we may find challenging and attempt to repress in some way. It is very relevant here, because as we journey to find peace in stillness, we may feel scared of what may come up in these quiet, dark times.

Somewhere in our shadows, for many of us who find it so hard to be still, is a distrust of ourselves, an insidious belief that if we were

In our 'water hours,' it is thought to be most beneficial to be calm in body and mind. So this might be another time you can embrace as time for dark magic.

to stop and rest we would fall into a pit of laziness and inaction, and never again achieve anything!

All of us have elements of ourselves that we don't like, or think society won't like, so we brush them into our subconscious minds. This is what Jung referred to as our shadow self. Healing can occur when we delve into these elements of our subconscious. However, we are often not fully aware of those shadows, distancing ourselves psychologically from behaviours, emotions and thoughts that we find challenging.

Seeing the shadows within ourselves can be extremely difficult. The mind tends to ignore these shadows to protect itself. And so what we often do instead is pick up on these 'flaws' in others – Jung calls this projection. While our conscious minds are avoiding our own shadows, they still want to deal with them on a deeper level, so we may pick out these behaviours in others (just like when I notice students unable to relax in meditation, knowing I'm just the same!)

Our conscious awareness is like a spotlight, allowing us to observe what is happening inside our minds. Beneath that conscious 'light' is a whole world of 'darkness' containing aspects of ourselves that we may strive to ignore. Our unconscious mind is an unseen shadow of our persona beneath our awareness, secretly guiding much of what we say, think and do.

When we apply how Jung uses the words "light" and "darkness" here, we might find that we are using actions and busy-ness, our visible persona and yang side, to perhaps cover the shadows we may find in the darkness and stillness of yin. The proposed solution is to do 'shadow work': the process of bringing the unconscious into the light. We can begin this process by taking a step back from our typical behaviour patterns and observe what is happening within us. Meditation and yin yoga are a great way to cultivate this ability to 'step back', and from here we may take the idea of *svadhyaya* (a yogic term meaning introspection and study of self) to pause, explore and question: "Why am I reacting in this way?"

The aim is not to defeat the shadow self: this is not a battle. Rather our intention is to weave together all facets of ourselves, not fear our shadows as we reach for wholeness.

You may find nighttime, and other times of dark are conducive to connecting to your shadow self. If you suffer from anxiety, depression and/or overwhelm I strongly suggest seeking help to work with your shadows from a qualified counsellor or therapist. You do not need to fear the dark, but you also don't have to journey through it alone. Treat yourself with care.

NIGHT

Yin's soft, nurturing, and passive energy is supported by the darkness and quiet of the night. And in turn, the night is defined in her yin qualities of darkness and stillness. *Shen* energy functions in the day and rests during the night to allow the organs and meridians to rest and recharge. Aggravated *shen* can affect how we sleep. Spirit, as you may imagine, can be disturbed by devices, working late, arguing and stress. I am personally terrible for staying up too late, looking at my phone in bed for an hour and then, unsurprisingly, being unable to switch off my mind and sleep when I do turn the lights off. But on days where I do manage to ditch my devices and read or practice yoga before bed, gently winding down as the day's light dims, I notice how much better I sleep.

Sleeping is a very yin activity, so sleeping during this yin period helps the body rejuvenate more fully (as opposed to, say, people who party all night and sleep in the day). When we are in tune with the rhythm of the earth, our sleep is deeper and sweeter.

YIN YOGA FOR SLEEP

Here are some yin yoga poses that can help nourish your yin energy and soothe your inner fire, by connecting to the meridians of Water (Kidneys/Bladder) and Earth (Spleen/Stomach) – to help you to journey towards peaceful sleep. Stay in each pose for 3-5 minutes if that's comfortable for you. (As always, head to sentiayoga.com/yin-magic to see these poses and more.)

Shoelace

You may know this position from hatha yoga, as Cow Face Pose.

From seated, bend your knees and put the soles of your feet on the earth. Bring your left foot under the right knee to the outer right hip. Cross your right leg over the left, stacking the right knee on top of the left; the right foot comes to the outside of the left hip. The shape of your legs is intended to represent the cow, your stacked knees are the nose, and your feet are the ears! Sit evenly on the sitting bones, resting your hands on your feet. Breathe and settle here. You can stay upright, or work into a forward fold if you like. Repeat on the other side.

Waterfall

From lying on your back, bring a cushion underneath your hips and lower back, creating a tilt in the pelvis towards your head. From here you can gently raise the legs to the sky. If this feels too challenging, you can do this same pose with your legs running up a wall for extra support.

To create a stretch through the hips for connection to the Kidney/Bladder meridian you can open the legs into a straddle (wide legs) for a minute or two.

Savasana

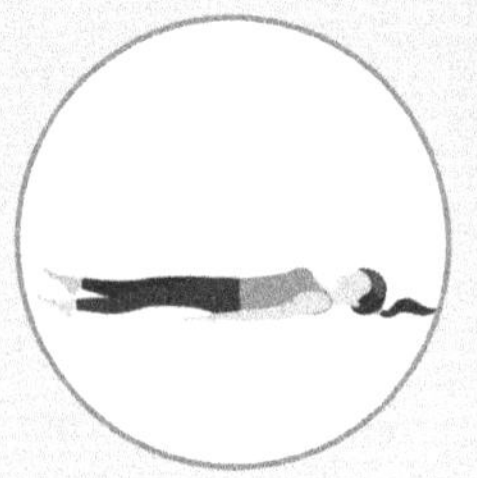

Roll back down to lay flat on the ground in Relaxation Pose, with a pillow or bolster under the knees. And let the body, mind and breath settle to calm.

Simple Sleeping Spell

Some herbal magic for a blissful night's sleep.

You will need:

- ☾ *Small cotton bag*
- ☾ *Traditional Western herbs often used for calming: dried lavender, chamomile and rose petals*
- ☾ *And/or Traditional Chinese herbs for calming: dried lotus seeds and willow bark*
- ☾ *And/or Ayurvedic herbs for grounding: nutmeg and cardamom*
- ☾ *Essential oils: lavender, Roman chamomile and clary sage*
- ☾ *Crystals: selenite, amethyst and/or hematite*
- ☾ *Clear intention*

(You can interchange any of these elements as you require.)
Place your herbs in a bowl or cauldron, mix them all together, put your mixture in your bag, and add your crystals as well. Carefully add three drops of each of your oils to the bag. Shake your bag, and it can go under your pillow or hang it by your bed.

NEW MOONS

Most nights are dark, but nights of the new moon, are the darkest, most yin of all.

Every month the moon moves into the same constellation as the sun. This lunar-solar meeting is what we call a new moon. New moons are a time for beginnings, stillness and introspection, a time to sit with shadows and ourselves.

The moon, throughout its journey of orbiting the earth each lunar month, spends a little over two days passing through each zodiac sign[ii]. This means that each month the moon's new phase coincides with a different zodiac sign, each with its own element and seasonal attributes. We also have 'seasons' of each zodiac sign, known as our birth sign.

While the new moon is in each sign, we may feel its energy (and potentially more so if it is your birth sign). All new moons are a great time to make plans, particularly for the next six months, after which the full moon will rise in the same sign, completing a cycle of our journey.

Of course, there are many other astrological variables at play at any time, such as the year and the positions of the other planets, particularly Jupiter, Venus, and Mercury. But this is a starting point to consider the sign of each new moon and the kind of yin-tastic new moon magic you may wish to explore.

☾ *For more on astrology and moon magic, I can recommend the fabulous websites of Chani Nicholas (chaninicholas.com) and Yasmin Boland (yasminboland.com) which are full of information and free resources.*

☾ *The specific date for new moons varies each year, but the cycle of the zodiac months remains the same. Southern hemisphere variations of seasons can be found at sentiayoga.com/yinmagic*

Winter New Moons

The new moons in the dark months of the year bring an extra dose of yin. This is a time of dark moons in cold, dark seasons: Yule and Imbolc. We learn that the dark is not something to fear, but something

ii Many cultures have astrological systems based on the movements of the planets, sun and moon and their correlation to stars. In this chapter I'll be drawing on the modern Western twelve sign zodiac.

within which we can find our stillness and our strength: time for turning inwards, both physically and spiritually. In this quiet time, we can make our plans for the coming year, and reflect on what we have achieved so far. Just as nature is resting, it is an excellent time to enjoy rest, and cosy evenings by the fire. Spells, rituals and yoga practice around this time may explore release and letting go, washing away like water.

1. New Moon in Capricorn

Sign: Earth **Months:** December to January
Season: Winter

In the Northern Hemisphere, we are in the darkest time of year. So, when the new moon comes along, we're in the deepest dark: winter and shadow. Take time to make your plans with care and balance. A plan of baby steps can help guide you towards more expansive journeys and transformation even when you cannot see the light.

2. New Moon in Aquarius

Sign: Air **Months:** January to February
Season: Winter

Aquarians walk their path in their own stride and have a unique sense of self. During this new year/new moon combination, we may find ourselves drawn towards radical transformation. This can be a time to honour change – just as the Taoists do – not work against it. Allow yourself to connect to your unique ideas and give them time to take root before letting others judge or comment, as these delicate dreams can be easily trampled.

3. New Moon in Pisces

Sign: Water **Months:** February to March
Season: Winter/Spring

The watery sign of Pisces could be thought of as a stream of healing and inspiration, of waters that wash away and reveal what's hiding beneath the surface. Every new moon is a time of rebirth – a time when we are given a chance to start afresh. Explore goals that embrace the kind, receptive, and dreamy energies of Pisces. Take time for peaceful, rejuvenating activities, which may include yoga and meditation.

Spring New Moons

The nights are beginning to shorten as the light of spring creeps in. The seasons of Ostara and Beltane bring light and a little extra warmth! This is a time to unravel, unfurl like a flower bud: have a good stretch and reawaken! It's time to clean out your home and heart. Open the windows to let in the scent of the spring awakening. This is a time to grow: spells, rituals and yoga practice around this time may explore the growth and fertility in all things in your life from new families and relationships to new projects and adventures.

4. New Moon in Aries

Sign: Fire
Months: March to April
Season: Spring

Aries carries with it raw qualities of beginnings – a force powerful enough to announce spring, and energy that breaks through the barrier of winter to begin again. Seek the courage to leave the past behind, and birth something different. Be brave and fearless in your intentions, write them all down before your inner critic has a chance to stop you.

5. New Moon in Taurus

Sign: Earth
Months: April to May
Season: Spring

Taurus is a sign of seeking comfort, groundedness, pleasure and indulgence. The Taurus new moon is a time to connect to the earthy magic of green witchery, making practical magic such as preparing soil and planting seeds for luscious food and flowers.

6. New Moon in Gemini

Sign: Air **Months:** May to June
Season: Spring

Embracing Gemini energy at new moon is about connecting to your desires and harmonizing the threads of your path. Meditation and mindfulness are ideal for air signs. As an air sign myself, my mind is prone to wander, and ideas can get lost! Meditation helps me draw back my focus. Pay attention to your words: spoken, written, and thought. Communication is especially important during this lunar phase. It's time to explore your inner dialogue. Words are powerful, so write your intentions in a journal or speak your wishes aloud in spell or ceremony.

Summer New Moons

The lightest and warmest nights are with us now. On the Wheel of the Year we are passing through Litha, Midsummer and Lammas celebrations. It is the season to go forth and bound into the light! Celebrate your full growth in this season: get outside, move and rejoice in the sun and laughter of being with loved ones. Spells, rituals and yoga practice around this time may explore abundance and joy. Feel empowered to strengthen and build upon this summer energy.

7. New Moon in Cancer

Sign: Water **Months:** June to July
Season: Summer

Cancer, as a water sign, represents the feminine, the moon and intuition. As we enter summer, this new moon can bring high energy and raw emotions to the surface. Allow yourself to cry, shout or scream should you need to. Sit with your grief, anger or sadness; you may want to keen, sing or drum with your emotions. Allow yourself space to work through your feelings. As we move forward into summer, the more we honour the rhythmicity in our lives, the stronger we become. If you need to rest, rest. If you need to howl at the moon, then do!

8. New Moon in Leo

Sign: Fire **Months:** July to August
Season: Summer

Leo is a fire sign, so within the energy of this new moon is a chance to be bold, make sparks and plans that help you to shine. You might make big changes and scrap all the plans that don't bring you joy. Throw out your old ideas and start all over again, thanking your path for all you have learned as you prepare to dance down a new road lined in summer flowers!

9. New Moon in Virgo

Sign: Earth **Months:** August to September
Season: Summer

The symbol of Virgo is the earth maiden; she loves to heal and provide. You may be guided toward restorative or healing work in order to allow you to give more to others (wise Virgo knows you cannot pour from an empty cup). Look at what you can add to your life to allow it to run more smoothly and drop elements that drain or stress you.

Autumn New Moons

As we move into the seasons of Mabon and Samhain the harvest brings joy to the journey towards the darker season. This is the time to gather in and surrender to the dark once more, a time to reflect and prepare to let go of the past year. Enjoy harvesting what you have grown through the warmer seasons, whether that be intentions or crops from your garden! Spells, rituals and yoga practice around this time may explore gratitude and grounding.

10. New Moon in Libra

Sign: Air **Months:** September to October
Season: Autumn

This new moon has an energetic focus on balance, harmony and social interactions. Are you finding your balance? Or have you been giving more than you have been receiving? Take time to reconnect with your personal balance. Work with green candles and use rose and bergamot essential oils to dress them. Call forth energies to open the heart chakra for balance and connection with the universe.

11. New Moon in Scorpio

Sign: Water
Months: October to November
Season: Autumn

Scorpio is the sign of the occult because it is the zodiac sign during Samhain and Halloween, and is represented by the image of the deadly scorpion. This is a powerful time for working with ideas of death, memory, intuition and the afterlife. You may want to create an altar or offerings to your ancestors. Consider scrying, divination and working with grounding crystals, focusing on your inner world or working with dark goddesses. Shadows and the dark goddesses aren't evil, they're just another aspect of who we are, just like the dark moon phase itself. This is a time for witches to embrace their shadows and their darkness.

12. New Moon in Sagittarius

Sign: Fire
Months: November to December
Season: Autumn/winter

Sagittarius is a sign between seasons: crossing over from autumn to winter. This may be a time to shake loose energy and set down baggage in preparation for a new journey. Take time to grow, learn and ignite new ideas and knowledge. You may ask questions of yourself such as: What is my vision for the future? How can I connect to healing and balance? Consider creating a dream or vision board for what you yearn to bring to fruition. Give yourself room to move through ideas, to wander through dreams, to see life through fresh eyes, and find bridges and doorways to connect your journey with some deeper meaning.

Slow Spell – Dark Moon Oil Infusion

The new moon is a special time for cultures in both East and West – we bring together the five elements here in this slow spell for balance and harmony. A beautiful spell to start on a dark night, this slow oil infusion takes two lunar cycles. You can start on a quiet night, and you will work with it as the power develops through the weeks. I'll outline the basic spell below, which can be tailored to your specific practice and intentions.

It uses a synergistic blend of herbs and spices that are easy to buy dried. Because we have been exploring the idea of the elements in the Chinese system, these herbs are also ones that connect to the five wu xing elements.

For the Oil Base:

Sweet almond oil: this is the oil I always use because it supports the prosperity of the spell.

(Kitchen Witch Note: If you wanted to use the oil in cooking, try olive oil or avocado oil as your base. The clove and cinnamon will dominate the flavour so use sparingly, or adjust the herbs – fennel and rosemary are a delicious pairing on their own).

Herbs and spices

Use dried herbs, as moisture can shorten the life of the oil.

Fennel – Representing the element of earth – this herb is for courage and standing strong.

Lavender – Representing the element air and the moon – this herb is for peace.

Rosemary – Representing the element of water – for love and clarity.

Cinnamon – Representing the element of fire – my favourite folklore of the cinnamon tree is that the phoenix builds its nest from the spicy cinnamon branches. Cinnamon in magic represents fresh starts and picking ourselves up from the ashes. It can support us in releasing what no longer serves us.

Clove – Representing the element of metal – for abundance and healing.

To infuse the oil:

1. *Fill a glass jar with your desired herbs and spices. Use a generous pinch of each. Call in the energy of each element (or what you wish to draw from each elemental energy) as you add it to the jar. You may also use the zodiac sign of the new moon to guide and inspire your intentions.*
2. *Cover the herbs with the oil – which is our connecting element. You can place the jar on your altar during this time, or in any cool, dark place.*
3. *Each week sit with the jar, shake it up and focus on the herbs as they settle, when they have become still, hopefully, you will also feel more still. If you are working towards manifestation, you may call on what you are hoping to manifest during this stilling practice.*
4. *Let the mixture infuse for two lunar cycles. When it has infused, you can leave the herbs in the oil or strain the infusion, depending on what you want to use it for.*
5. *Use it at the new moon. You may wish to use it to anoint a candle or yourself or add it to a bath – this will be personal to your practice.*

WINTER

Winter in many parts of the world is a season of bitter cold, snow and long nights. Yin reaches its height of influence at winter solstice (around the 21st December in the Northern hemisphere and the 21st June in Southern Hemisphere).

The months leading up Samhain and the last harvest were once a time of planning and preparation. Extra food was prepared: vegetables and fruits canned and stored, wood gathered and seasoned for the hearth fires. Now winter food and warmth are less scarce, but if you listen to the rhythm of nature, it is still a natural time to draw inwards, prepare and find a slower pace. This is a great time to meditate on the past year and what it has meant to you. If there is something which has affected you strongly, this would be a good time to do a spell for letting go or releasing the emotions it produced.

Winter is also a great time to catch up on things like connecting with family. Give thanks for everything that has made you who you are – the ancestors, the lessons you have learned, the time you have enjoyed with loved ones. Many witches will have just started a new year after Samhain so take some time and think about what you want this new year to be. Perhaps it is to be a year of adventure or of self-care and recovery? Would you like to learn more about divination, blending oils, or other magical workings? The slower pace of winter is the perfect time to think about it and to start to gather what you will need. Wrap up warm and take a long winter's walk. Study the new landscapes and shape of nature in this season as it, like you, recharges and reflects. Whatever you love to do, the slower pace of winter can give you the time to do it.

Winter is full of festivities and parties and events to bring light, cheer and brighten the dark days and nights, and it is lovely to embrace these festive elements. But you should also connect and listen to what your body and mind want during the winter season – which may well be a slower pace. You may instinctually feel a desire to withdraw, slow down, and rest. However, the modern world often demands us to keep up with our work schedules and obligations regardless of the cold, black darkness outside. To listen to your own energy levels is a yin rebellion and an invitation to challenge popular ideas about constant doing. Withdrawing your energy from something is an act of resistance to the status quo, it is also a wise choice because our energy is finite. When we take time to rest, reflect and assess where our energy is going, we may see that if we try and 'do it all' we will inevitably fail in some area. It's about trusting yourself to do what is important to you, but also in letting go of what isn't.

The Call of the Dark Goddess

From Mabon until Ostara is the reign of the dark goddesses of autumn and winter. You may feel the presence of the winter goddesses in the air and see them in the beauty of the snowfall and icicles.

To meet a winter goddess, spend time in meditation or reading cards. Be open to learning about her culture and to feeling her energy: she may have words, insight or wisdom for you. Celebrate this yuletide and winter season in your own way and be sure to honour your own rhythms and what the dark goddess calls to within you. (I'll talk more about specific goddesses of the dark, winter and of yin in the next chapter).

Flame Gazing

Pyromancy is divination through gazing upon the flames of your candle. If you have a fireplace, you can gaze into these flames too. Hold a question or guidance you are seeking in your mind, see what comes to mind or what images dance in the flames. Burning petitions or offerings for spellwork can also be useful and beautiful.

Find a Light

Lighting candles is a simple and powerful way of creating a personal connection to the light, like that little spot of white in the dark yin side of the yin yang symbol. It is also a connection to your ancestors, who would have lit candles each day by necessity, to bring light to the dark.

Candle magic is an ancient form of sympathetic magic. Candles are used in rituals to represent people, things, and emotions. Casting a spell focuses one's intent to influence the desired outcome represented by the candle.

Coloured candles are used for their symbolic correspondences. The correspondences below are drawn from various alchemical and astrological resources, which may vary depending on your school of thought and own intuition.

- Red signifies courage, health and passion. (Aries).
- Pink signifies friendship and love.
- Purple signifies power, spirituality and meditation. (Virgo).
- Yellow signifies protection, success and attraction. (Gemini).
- Orange signifies encouragement, attraction and adaptability.
- Gold signifies success, the sun's energy and abundance. (Leo).
- Blue signifies health, knowledge and patience. (Aquarius, Pisces and Sagittarius).
- Green signifies fertility and abundance. (Libra and Taurus).
- Black signifies healing and transformation. (Scorpio).
- White signifies truth, protection and peace. (Cancer).
- Brown is related to the earth goddesses, elementals and animals. (Capricorn).
- Silver signifies intuition and lunar connections.

You may wish to anoint the candle with essential oil. If your goal is to draw something toward you, anoint from the ends of the candle inwards to the middle. To repel something, rub from the centre to the ends.

You may also wish to use a chant or mantra like the following:

Element of Fire, I call upon you
Candle of power, let magic pass through you
.......[iii]
My words have strength; this spell is done.
Do as ye will, and harm ye none.

iii You can add any specific intentions or wishes you may have here.

MENSTRUATION

When we are speaking of embracing the dark, I can't leave out what was once a sacred time, traditionally a time to isolate and rest: menstruation. This is another kind of connection/synchronisation with darkness and light, yin and yang. The moon also plays a vital role here, as women's cycles have long been connected to the cycles of the moon, as well as to the waxing and waning of waters, and other women as we entrain to each others' cycles.

Ritual and menstruation share ancient connections. The term 'ritual' is derived from the Sanskrit word *r'tu*, which refers to both sacred times and menstruation. This idea that some of the earliest rituals would have been in connection to woman's monthly bleeding has, to many, been lost in time (or purposefully discarded). And while it may be hard to see this time as a sacred blessing (especially for those of us who experience pain and discomfort), perhaps we can at least begin to turn away from the stereotype of it being a 'curse'.

In many ancient cultures, women would separate themselves while menstruating for reasons ranging from fear to reverence. Stepping away from the yang of family responsibilities and entering the sacred realms of yin: quiet time to rest, dream, nurture and possibly receive spiritual insight. The restful dark allowed renewal of wisdom and purpose.

There was certainly an air of 'dark magic' about this time, a mystery and 'otherness' as women disappeared from day-to-day life. In some of these cultures it was believed that women created a channel to the sacred mysteries of life and death, and menstruation was a proof of this magic. It is easy to see how it all got woven together up with the occult and esotericism…and then became despised and unspeakable once matrifocal practices were displaced by patriarchal ones.

Energy ebbs and flows differently during menstruation, so listening to your body is key; many crave rest and stillness at this time. We may not be able to fully retreat for a week, but it may be a time to treat yourself with more yin compassion and practice sacred care. As the revolution of the rising feminine grows in our culture, there is a recognised need to come back to some of these ideas.[iv] You will find moon lodges and red tents are now held in many cities and countries, where women can gather and celebrate the powerful and intuitive times of their own energies and cycles. Visit redtentdirectory.com to find one near you.

R'tu

Many Sanskrit words have a variety of meanings, but r'tu is a beauty for a selection of power words! R'tu means, amongst other things: season, menstruation, light, splendour, appointed time, right action, epoch.
R'tu is also the root word for rtusandhi – days of the new and full moon, and k'Rta and k'Rti meaning magic!

DARK YOGA

While many yin sequences draw on the wisdom of the meridians, using 'dark' themes for our yin yoga is another way to celebrate them as special and sacred, a time to be enjoyed! The beauty of weaving together the ideas of the witch and the yogi is that we can weave magic and healing in so many ways. Yin yoga is a practice that can soothe an aching body during menstruation, calm and focus the mind at new moon, bring comfort and grounding if needed on a dark stormy night, aid sleep or simply to embrace a quiet evening.

These yin sequences can be used anytime you feel the need to cultivate more yin for yourself. I invite you to explore the connection between yin yoga and times of magical significance to deepen your journey towards yin magic.

iv From redtentdirectory.com: Red tents are open to "women-identified and non-binary femme of centre people. In other words, if you need a safe and brave space to connect with feminine wisdom, power, and nurturing, this circle is for you, whether you have a menstrual cycle or not."

Nighttime and new moons are regular reminders and invitations to find our yin, so these sequences are named after these yin times. (I'll outline the poses briefly here and, as always, further details, images and videos can be found at sentiayoga.com/yinmagic).

NEW MOON YIN SEQUENCE

Melting Heart

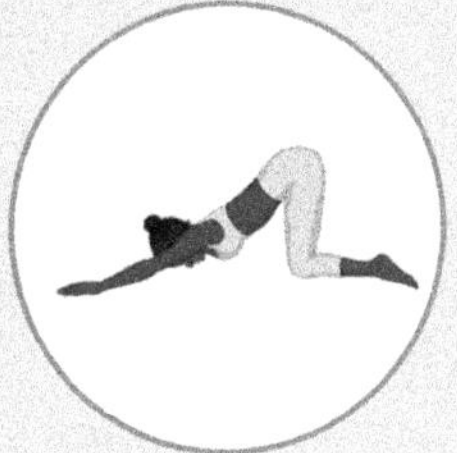

From all fours, slide the hands forward and rest your forehead on the earth, shining your heart towards the ground.

Melting Heart Twist

From Melting Heart, slide your right hand under your left armpit so you are resting on the right shoulder and right side of the head, to create a twist in the upper back. The left hand can stay reaching towards the top of your mat, or can be wrapped behind your body to your right hip like a spiral thread (pictured).

Happy Baby

Lying on your back, draw your knees in towards your armpits, opening through the hips. Shining the soles of the feet to the sky, hold the outer edges of the feet. If this feels too much, you can do Half Happy Baby, holding onto the knees, drawing them in toward your armpits.

Bananasana

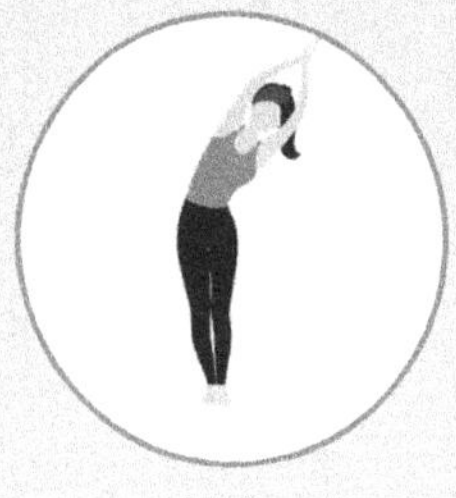

From lying on the ground (this image is a top view!) the crescent moon shape opens through the side of the body.
Optional ending: *savasana* (lying on the back) for meditation.

NIGHTTIME YIN SEQUENCE

Caterpillar/Forward Fold

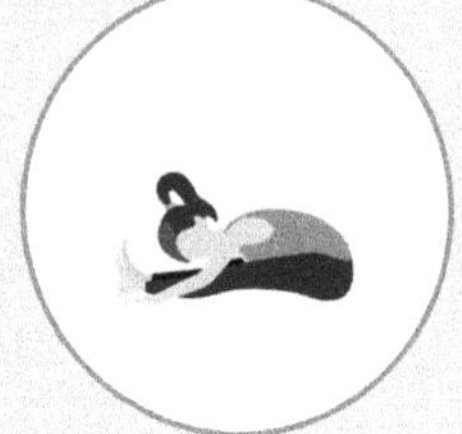

From seated with extended legs, fold forwards, hinging from the hips. Let the head hang heavy like the sun drifting towards the horizon.

Child's Pose

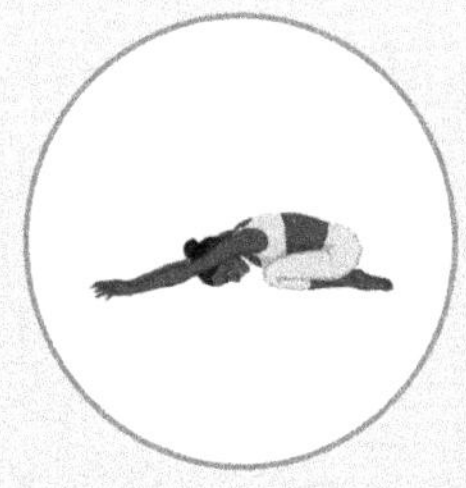

From all fours drop the bum down upon the heels and reaching your hands forward, rest your forehead upon the earth. Bring in cushions for extra support if needed, you can have knees wide or narrow depending on what's most restful for you.

Reclining Twist

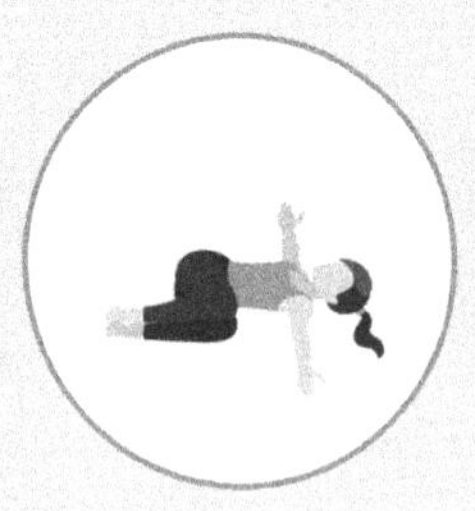

Lying on your back, bend your knees and rest the soles of the feet on the floor. Arms can settle wide on the earth. Let the knees fall to right and the gaze can go to the left in a gentle and passive spiral twist. Settle and relax. Repeat on other side.

Supported Bridge

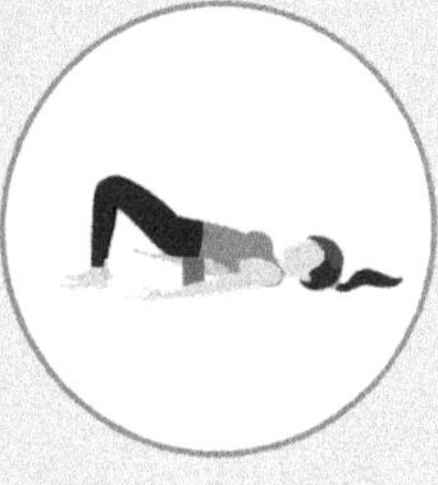

From lying on your back, bend the knees and bring the soles of the feet on the floor. Lift the hips gently and bring a support under the hips in the form of a cushion or bolster.

Reclining Butterfly

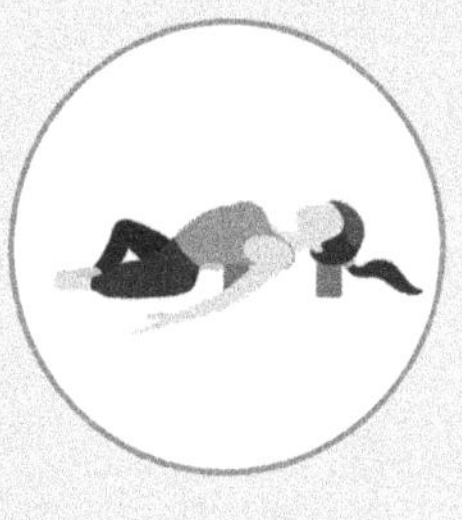

Soles of the feet come together and the knees fall out on either side like a butterfly's wings (this image shows where you may want to bring in support in the form of pillows, but it's not essential. You may prefer to settle on the earth).

Move into lying flat on the earth, *savasana* ready for sleep/meditation.

Corpse Pose

Savasana actually means pose of the corpse. Death may well be another place of 'dark' that may illicit trepidation and fear. But just as when we slip into sleep, we are simply slipping into a new realm of consciousness, each time we move into the pose of the corpse in yoga practice we are offered a chance to let go and be reborn!

YIN MANIFESTATION

We can use these yin ideas and dark times to bring new energy to our manifestation spellwork.

I think manifestation is a great place to draw the ideas of the yin feminine into mind. Because manifestation – if approached from a yang, masculine standpoint – can become like a shopping list, focused more on what you want from the universe than how you are looking to change and grow as a person. Manifestation is not a trolley-dash for desires, but a mindful journey, a steady process of self-study, growth and change. And while I definitely talk about seeking goals and dreams, its useful to remember that these should really be way-markers on the journey. They are not the endpoint.

The process of conjuring the vision of our path at the new moon, and then seeing the process through to the light of our biggest dreams, is a significant undertaking. One that needs to be done in conscious stages. It ensures that we take time to not only harvest the seeds we have sown but to leave time for rest: just as nature rests in winter so that we have the energy to prepare for the next steps on our journey.

We live in a culture where waiting for anything has become almost obsolete – if we want a book, film, recipe, we can have it in moments, with a few clicks on a screen. It can be hard to remember that we as humans cannot work to this same instant timeline: our work takes longer. But still we cram our days with huge to-do lists in the name of peak productivity, and then feel guilt and shame that we have been unable to keep up with this fast pace. We often run through days and still feel like we have not 'done enough'.

There is no 'enough', there is no 'perfect'. So if you can, try and let go of your ideas of how much you should produce, and prioritise slowing down. Let your mind wander. Give yourself time to incubate and nurture seedlings of ideas. And give yourself free time, like these dark evenings, with no grand, intricate plan. You cannot schedule in 'inspiration' like a meeting. If you do, you may find that you experience blocks or even feel that you are not creative: you are, I promise! But it's something that needs time, patience, and a little rebel spirit to fly in the face of instant gratification. Allow yourself to work instead with slow and mindful inspiration, enjoying and savouring each step of the journey, accepting the steps you make, no matter how small.

So this outline is about finding a balance between our yang drive to succeed and share, and our yin needs to slow down and be still so that we can be true to and honour ourselves and the journey.

I'd love to help you towards finding the inner '*yuj*' – the yoking of our yin and yang sides, between being and doing, receiving and giving. Constantly throwing out requests to the universe and a striving for 'more' can leave you feeling tired and discouraged, so let's look at how we can consciously and sustainably move into manifesting magic. Take time to cycle through each of these four stages of manifestation, to help nurture the sparks of your dreams and desires, to focus, to prioritise, to be prepared to work and journey and not burn out!

1. The Dream (New Moon)

This is the most yin stage of creation. The dream season is winter and the new moon phase. We hold the spark of insight within us. Maybe you call it a vision, intuition, dream or an invisible nudge from deep inside. Trust in these tiny sparks, connect and listen to them. They will answer, if you slow down, get quiet, and give them the space to whisper to you.

2. The Seed (Waxing Moon)

This is where yin and yang start to intermingle and unite. Seed season is spring and Imbolc, and the waxing moon phase. The energy of life is ready to spring forth. So much growth happens during this stage, but only at a very tiny level. The seed is still hidden underground, nurture it gently in the dark earth.

3. The Bloom (Full Moon)

Now yang takes the lead. The season is summer, the element of fire and the moon phase is full. Once the seed bursts from the earth, it's up and out: growing, blossoming, moving ahead, clearing the path. There's rapid growth and partnership here, arriving in the full light of day for all to see and partake in – this corresponds to the execution and embodiment of our vision.

4. The Harvest (Waning Moon)

Yin and yang blend together once more. This is the time to slow down, reflecting while harvesting. The correspondences to this phase are the season of autumn and the waning moon. After the blooms we have created, it's time to quieten and reflect. What did you learn from the process? What was successful? What can you do differently next time? Harvest the fruits you have grown from seed, receive them with gratitude.

We need each of these stages. Not rushed, but one at a time. Like the seasons, lunar cycles and ocean waves, this cycle, this rhythm, rolls over and over again in endless, unhurried, creative phases.

CLOSING YINSIGHTS

Once it would have been prudent for our survival to avoid dark caves, dark corners and to be fair, that's probably still wise! But we need not fear all darkness! The dark can represent the unknown and unknowable, but within ourselves there is an opportunity within the dark to know ourselves a little better and connect with ourselves in more meaningful ways. I encourage you to take sanctuary in the dark, and the magic therein. If you need a little more help to embrace the yin dark – then perhaps the goddesses of the next chapter may offer some inspiration…

9

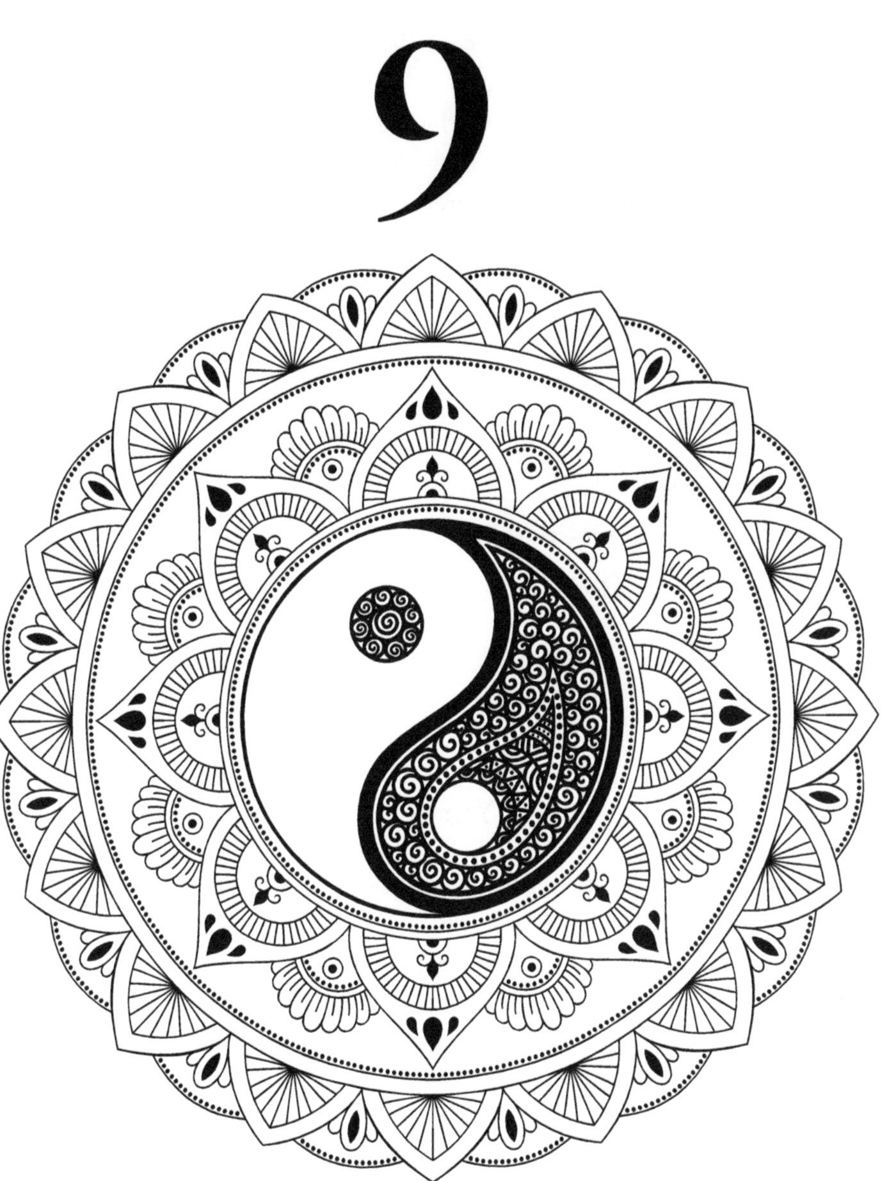

GODDESSES OF YIN

Welcome to just some of the goddesses I am naming the Goddesses of Yin, because of their corresponding elements of winter, nighttime, the moon and the element of water. If we are to delve into yin and find stillness and a certain magic, then these special Goddesses of Yin surely may have something to teach us.

Our Goddesses:

1. Kuan Yin (Chinese)
2. Jiu Tian Xuan Nu – The Dark Goddess of the Ninth Heaven (Chinese)
3. Parvati (Hindu)
4. Akhilandeshvari – The Goddess of Never Not Broken (Hindu)
5. Beira (Celtic/Gaelic)
6. Angerona (Roman)
7. Kerridwen (Celtic)

Kuan Yin (Chinese)

Kuan Yin has to come above all others in a book about the magic of yin – it's in her name after all. The yin in her name is the yin of listening, kindness and compassion.

But first a confession: she's not actually a goddess… Kuan Yin, as a bodhisattva, is mortal-born. A bodhisattva is a being of enlightenment that could have ascended to be a Buddha but chooses to stay on earth and help humanity reach enlightenment. This is in no way a discouragement to petition or seek guidance from Kuan Yin. As a bodhisattva, she is connected to the divine, one step away from becoming a deity – but at the threshold of heaven, she chooses to stay and to help us.

And help us she does: to connect to our abilities to be self-compassionate, something in itself that has, to some, come to mean a kind of weakness. Society often suggests that to be gentle and kind is some sort of luxury we can do without (we've all heard sayings like "no pain no gain" and "failure is not an option"). This could not be more wrong. In empirical studies, students were more likely to perform better in tasks if they had previously been encouraged to practice self-compassion towards earlier failures. People who practice self-compassion are less afraid to fail: understanding failures instead as an opportunity to learn and grow.

We will all fail at multiple times throughout our lives: from small accidents like forgetting to check on the oven and burning the brownies or despite our best efforts, failing to make a new business venture work. This is not intended to distress, just to illustrate that it is unavoidable. It is a part of life. But in being self-compassionate, we are less scared of trying new things lest we fail. There is a bravery in self-compassion, in allowing yourself to be as you are.

Jiu Tian Xuan Nu – The Dark Goddess of the Ninth Heaven (Chinese)

In Chinese myth there are nine layers of heaven and The Dark Goddess – sometimes translated as The Mysterious Lady of the Ninth Heaven – presides over them all. Taoists depict her with a sword in her right hand. In her left hand, she holds a gourd: a symbol of immortality, healing and longevity. She rides a phoenix, dressed in gowns made of the colours of bird feathers. She taught emperors the art of war in cosmic battles, gifting mortals texts on alchemy, healing magic and immortality. She's a deity of the occult arts, magic and spellcraft, as well as strength, power and health.

The deity of Taoist sorcery, she would have been petitioned in the quest of the alchemist to find eternal life. Alchemy, with its many definitions, means among other things, to rise to one's fullest potential. For humans (according to alchemists) this was eternal life or enlightenment and for base metals it was to become gold. Jiu Tian Xuan Nu may be considered a deity to help us rise with our own alchemy of becoming – to become our best and truest selves, reaching our fullest potential according to our own values and our most harmonious life.

She could be compared to a benevolent spirit and holds Kuan Yin in high esteem, but she is a very different goddess. I consider her almost like the dot of yang within the yin symbol. Or the yang dawn at the end of the yin night: she is the bringer of the daylight gate, the point of crossing over.

To me, Jiu Tian Xuan Nu represents yang self-compassion in harmony with Kuan Yin's yin self-compassion. Jiu Tian Xuan Nu is the goddess that supports us to say no, set boundaries and claim time for ourselves. Compassion isn't always yin and soft, sometimes it means being forceful. In yin self-compassion, we hold ourselves with love. In yang self-compassion, we act to protect ourselves with love. Acceptance and honouring of yourself as you are is part of this yang compassion. It is not always easy to show love to ourselves, but like all skills, it can be learnt, and we can improve with practice. You can learn what is right for you, and perhaps when to respectfully say no.

Working with the Dark Goddesses: Simple Shadow Work

Anoint yourself with your dark moon oil from Chapter 7 or light some incense. If you want to use traditional Chinese incense, you could choose Amber, Frankincense, Sandalwood, or Cedarwood.

Focus your attention – visualise all the many thoughts and stresses that are 'chasing you' or settled into your subconscious. And as you choose to turn and face these shadows, call out for the Dark Goddess of the Ninth Heaven and Kuan Yin to help you face your shadows, to see and acknowledge them.

Kuan Yin is watching over you and listening to you, and our dark goddess Jiu Tian Xuan Nu will stand beside you, to teach and inspire you to find the tools to journey forwards.

Parvati (Hindu)

Parvati is the goddess of love, beauty, divine strength and power. A representation of *shakti* – female energy, and she is relevant to anyone looking to balance strength with stillness.

Parvati becomes Durga

Durga is the warrior form of Goddess Parvati. The story begins with a powerful demon, who could not be beaten by god or man. Parvati – a great yogi and wife of god Shiva – volunteered herself to battle with the fearsome demon. To prepare for this challenge, Parvati secluded herself within a mountain cave to meditate. The gods sent her their best weapons for the fight that lay ahead, which is why we may see depictions of Parvati/Durga with many arms holding these gifts, including a bow and arrow signifying her grasp of both potential and dynamic energy (yin/yang and *shakti/shiva*).

Parvati's meditation before her battle shows the power of focus and the importance of stillness. Parvati takes on a terrifying commitment, and her first action is to slow down and give herself space to prepare: withdrawing in order to concentrate. She doesn't rush into busyness and does not flee. She understands the usefulness of stillness – the power of being before doing. This space for quiet focus is what gives her her incredible strength, receiving her divine resources. Pausing makes her strong, not weak, as she steels herself to face her enemies that may form as doubt, obstacles, or fatigue.

Parvati's transformation into Durga emphasises our own ability to connect to courage. Parvati is ultimately victorious; a reminder that sometimes courage looks like finding stillness when everyone around you is busy moving. Her victory was not trying to do everything at once or trying to meet the expectations of others; she had faith in herself and her ability to fulfil her powerful potential. Sometimes courage looks like choosing over and over again to honour your own *dharma*/path, and sometimes it is being willing to make mistakes and have doubts in your journey. There is a wonderful line of the Bhagavad Gita that says, "It is better to do one's own dharma, imperfectly, than to do another's dharma perfectly."

Walking in the Light of Dharma

Dharma is a term found in Buddhism, Hinduism and yoga. Dharma is not so much about 'success' but following the right path for you. In the self-study of our energy, we are seeking a path of harmony, balance and fulfilment. Our purpose is what makes us feel aligned, in flow and heartened, even when we make mistakes. Maybe finding our dharma allows us to release things we know are not for us. When we are lost, panicking, angry we may grasp at any offer, any project, hoping to find what is right. Whereas, and I think we know this deep down, the work has to start within. There may be a project that comes with a fancy title or lots of money, but if it is not your dharma, will you find peace and happiness on that path? Or stress and dis-ease? I think stillness can be found in the contentment of knowing you are on the right path, and knowing this path is a lifetime's work.

Akhilandeshvari (Hindu)

Ishvari in Sanskrit means goddess, queen or female power, and *Akhilanda* has a variety of Sanskrit translations such as "a collection of things" and "scattered pieces" but popular goddess translations have turned this into the enigmatic "never not broken."

This goddess is a representation of hurt and loss. When we experience extreme emotions or trauma we may describe ourselves as "going to pieces" or "falling apart." And so, this interpretation of the goddess who is "never not broken" is born.

While her exact name is open to some interpretation, her history has deep roots. She is a goddess from the ancient Hindu texts: the Vedas. She is also considered a form of Goddess Parvati and Durga. She carries a trident representing the three *gunas* and stands upon a crocodile upon a rushing river. (More threes! The three *gunas* are *tamas*, *rajas*, and *sattva*, attributes of inertia, action and harmony respectively.)

What is particularly exciting about Akhilandeshvari is that she derives her power not from being whole, but from being broken: from the pulling apart, like an atom that is split, releasing energy in what we call nuclear fission. If we travel back to Chapter 1 you will remember the Taoist origin story of *qi*, life force, as arising from the interaction between yin and yang. The yin and yang of Akhilandeshvari is here breaking apart and coming together. From this her power, her *qi*, is created.

Yin and yang are in constant flux and change, just like our goddess (and ourselves). Impermanence is the truth, the way, the Tao: of life, and of the human condition. Embracing it in can be the key to finding ease. This is a truth we may know in our minds but tend to resist in our hearts, which is another reason dark goddesses and goddesses connected to death are sometimes viewed with hesitation. Change is a constant in life, yet we long for the predictable reassurance that comes from things remaining the same.

The thing about going through sudden change or trauma is that it can destroy, for a time, our future: the story of our lives we had created in our minds about how things would unfold. What Akhilandeshvari offers us is the possibility and power of our choices from these broken pieces and uncertainty. Times when we are shifting and unfolding in new ways are a powerful opportunity to decide how we want to put ourselves back together. Confusion and unknowing are incredible teachers – no one has it all figured out; there is always a need to learn.

The goddess reminds us that with every new shiny whole we create, we will, one day, break apart once more and put ourselves together again in a perpetual cycle of life. But don't despair! In our brokenness, we are unlimited. We have the strength and ability to break, re-create and rebuild ourselves over and over.

Akhilandeshvari helps us to grow, to transform, to heal and to mend. She shows us how to embody the principle of *wu wei*, surrendering to the motion of life, the impermanence of reality, the flowing waters of the river, and the rhythm of nature, trusting that we will once again become a perfectly imperfect whole.

Beira (Celtic/Gaelic)

In Celtic myth Beira is also known as the Cailleach, Queen of Winter. The crone aspect of the Triple Goddess, ruler of the dark days of winter, she can be found in Ireland, Scotland and England, traced through folklore, ancient monuments, natural wonders, and stories.

As she rules the winter months, she embodies the Dark Mother, a kindly destroyer. As plants fall into stillness in late autumn, she appears as harvest goddess and the bringer of storms. In some depictions, Beira has just one eye, symbolising her ability to see beyond duality, and into the oneness of all beings – like the swirling yin-yang symbol all is encapsulated within this one circle.

In Celtic folklore, the wisdom of darkness is brought to life by powerful goddess figures. Goddesses like Beira helped bring hope to darkness, associating it with new beginnings: the potential of the seed below the ground. Their role was to ignite change through the transformative power of darkness, and to act as a guide through the process of death into new life. Many goddess figures bear strong similarities to the Cailleach/Beira in other European cultures such as Frau Holle (Germanic) and Baba Yaga (Slavic).

There are some myths that say that spring arrives when the crone goddess passes her mantle to Brigid, Goddess of Spring. Others say that on the longest night of the year, Beira marks the end of her reign as Queen of Winter by visiting the Well of Youth and, after drinking its magic water, grows younger day by day, becoming, in time, the Spring Maiden herself. She reaches full womanhood by summer and then returns through autumn to her form as crone. This is the triple goddess present in the natural world: maiden, mother and crone.

Angerona (Roman)

I've always been a fan of a good obscure Roman goddess. They all played their part in stories, myth and ancient culture, it's lovely to remember them. I named my yoga company after a little known Roman goddess called Sentia – the goddess who gifts beings with their sentience – which in turn connects to a common belief in nature-based religions of animism: that all things have energy and their own kind of sentience and spiritual essence, from plants and animals to crystals and elements.

Angerona's name may be drawn from the Latin roots *angustia* and *angor*, meaning difficulty or entanglement (our word "anguish" comes from it, as well as "anger"). She is the goddess of silence, secrets, and healing of fear, pain and sorrow. Some sources describe her as the goddess who not only produces anguish and fear within humans, but also relieves them from it. This is an interesting reflection of the need to feel and work through, in order to release emotion. With Angerona, to feel is also to be set free.

Her festival – Angeronalia – was celebrated in December, close to or on winter solstice, the darkest day of the year. The connection between darkness and silence may be why Angerona's festival was held at this time. Angerona helped guide both nature and humans through the darkest days, conjuring powerful magic to guide the sun to regain its strength.

In ancient Rome sacrifices were made to Angerona's statue in the temple of Volupia, the goddess of pleasure (interesting that this goddess of anguish is held in the temple of the pleasure goddess; emblematic perhaps of that we cannot have one without the other… and that working through these shadows will bring us to pleasure). In the temple of Volupia, the goddess Angerona was represented with her mouth bound and bandaged. In other depictions she has a finger pressed to her lips, demanding silence, hence my reasoning that she should be here amongst our goddesses of stillness and quiet power.

Silence does not merely refer to keeping secrets: silence can also be calming. Angerona's silence is of concentration and meditation. Her wisdom in silence is an encouragement to reflect on one's self and the world – an opportunity for clarity and healing. Angerona demands silence in times of crisis, dark midwinter and illness – a chance perhaps to pause and think. Silence is harder and harder to come by in today's busy world, hence the need for practices of meditation, mindfulness and yin yoga.

Winter Festivals

December was the end of the agricultural year and the beginning of winter for the Romans in Northern Europe. It was a busy month for festivals as they celebrated the harvest, as well as a warding against the darkness of winter, and made offerings to the gods in an attempt to ensure continued prosperity. (We still do some of this in winter, bringing many of our brightest and most jolly festivals into the darkest months from October lanterns, November bonfires and festivities, through to December fairy lights and January fireworks).

Winter festivals acknowledged a balance of both death, darkness, and reflection with celebration, joy and light. They marked both the stillness and silence of the season and a hopefulness for the return of the sun. As well as Angeronalia, during December, the Romans would have celebrated: Saturnalia to honour Saturn as the god of the harvest; the festival of Bona Dea (goddess of fertility); the Consualia (named after the god of grain); the Opalia (honouring Ops, the goddess of abundance and harvest); and the Larentalia (related to the underworld goddess, Acca Larentia, during which offerings were made to the dead).

Kerridwen (Celtic)

From Welsh medieval legend and Celtic mythology, Kerridwen, keeper of the cauldron is the great momma of making the most of the dark and embodying transformation in all its magical glory. She rules the realms of death, regeneration, magic and knowledge. Kerridwen continually stirs the spirals, the circles of life within her cauldron, symbol of the womb of the goddess where inspiration and divine knowledge swirl alongside the eternal cycle of birth, death and rebirth. Connection to Kerridwen is to invite change upon yourself, to see transformation is at hand. It is time to examine your life and recognise what no longer serves you, to embrace what must perish in order for something new and better to be born. Forging these fires of transformation will bring true inspiration into your life – change, growth and energy.

Kerridwen keeps a watch over all cauldrons (including our inner energy cauldrons as we explored in Chapter 5 – the Cauldrons of Warming, Vocation and Wisdom). Cauldrons would traditionally be made of iron, which interestingly is connected to Goddess Brigid in her connection to fire and forge (everything is connected, I know, it's magical!) Kerridwen has her own magical cauldron that holds potions of knowledge and inspiration. Those who taste of it will at once understand the secrets of creation – past, present and future. They will be transformed and reborn as eternally wise beings. Because of her great knowledge and insight, Kerridwen is almost always depicted as crone, and rightly so, as time and age are our greatest tools in gathering knowledge, experience and inspiration. Every day we learn and change a little more!

Like Angerona, she guards precious secrets. She has connections to the magic of divination, shaping and shifting. As a goddess of death and rebirth, Kerridwen stands at the crossroads, governing the underworld, reigning over the mysteries of life, death and transformation. She is the keeper of the gates between the worlds.

ON DARK GODDESSES

We imbue our emotions and traits onto our goddess archetypes, and goddesses of the night, winter, dark and crone form often get given, or administer, the 'shadow self' qualities such as anger, grief, sadness, uncertainty… Whilst these elements are an utterly natural part of our psyche, they are very often portrayed as things we should contain or suppress. Now I'm not saying anyone would want to be just these shadows, but they are needed… in balance with kindness, joy, gratitude, acceptance and patience.

As we explored in the previous chapter, shadow work can help us understand why we act a certain way, speak and feel as we do – exploring deeper into our own psyche. Meditation, journaling and divination are all tools we can use in union with the journey to explore what scares us, what are we suppressing and why.

This wild side of the Dark Goddess can be painted as this primal, evil force. And in humans when expressed, feelings like anger may be cast away and ignored as 'bad' instead of recognized, acknowledged and ultimately healed. But, and this is important: we all have a shadow self. And as women, we are often the ones that feel we need to cast these emotions into our unconscious or into hiding…which is why we often have a sympathy and a connection to the Dark Goddess as we face the struggles she has: the oppression, persecution, challenges, and feeling dismissed.

I like to think of the myth of Pandora and her jar of all the world's evils (often translated as a box) here. The name Pandora means "all gifts": *pan* = all, *doron* = gifts/treasures/giving. I don't think we focus on this nearly enough in the traditional telling of this tale, which is, quite irritatingly used more as a kind of reprimand to curious women. When in fact all Pandora, as the first woman forged by god Hephaestus, was doing, was creating the inevitable and essential balance in the world. After all, these 'evils' don't belong to the earth – greed, jealousy, anger – they are ours alone as humans. Maybe Pandora had to teach that to the gods…and to men. In order to experience all the gifts (the Pandora) of the human experience, one must experience all its sorrows as well. The emergence of hope, the last thing to leave the jar Pandora opens, helps support us on the journey. Despite it being portrayed as something tiny in the classic telling of the story, hope and belief are vital in harnessing the power of the psyche.

We struggle to deal with our shadow selves whether we form them as goddesses or not – but if we seek true peace, we cannot ignore them. And if we choose to do shadow work, we can use the help of the Dark Goddess to help light the way.

Care and Caution

Working with the Dark Goddess and shadow selves can be challenging if you have a history of issues such as depression or any physical or emotional trauma. Painful memories and emotions mean this work can be exhausting and challenging. So, if at any time you feel overwhelmed or triggered, or think you may do if working with shadows, please seek a professional and trusted teacher, counsellor or healer. The path to healing takes time. Blocks within our minds may exist to protect us. If you aren't ready to deal with these shadow elements yet, that's okay. This process can take months, years, a lifetime... and it is hard work. Try not to rush the process, and seek help when needed, or if you are just not sure.

Meditate with the Goddess

If you wish to, you can meet these goddesses in meditation. And they may form part of your work with your shadow self.

Take your time, as you journey inwards to meet these goddesses. Be patient and go slowly. There is no right or wrong way to connect to a goddess. You may want to float in stillness, journey with a drum, music or guided meditation. You might want to reflect on a goddess icon or image. You could draw or craft a goddess, read aloud a goddess mantra or create a shaker jar (see the boxed text). Observe and accept the thoughts and emotions that may be connected to the goddess or your own intuition. Let them arise without judgment. Every moment of stillness is an opportunity to learn and grow. Taking time to observe and notice your thoughts can help you nurture a more profound sense of presence and wellbeing.

Simple Shaker Jar Spell for Meditation

This super simple spell is for focus and stillness. You can have this jar on your altar, or even keep it with you in a pocket or bag.
You'll need:

- *A clean glass jar*
- *Dried mint for clarity of mind*
- *Dried rosemary for concentration*
- *Dried hawthorn to help you connect to the energy of your heart. Many cultures traditionally use hawthorn leaves and berries, including Native American, Chinese and European*

Other correspondence for specific yin goddesses

- *Kuan Yin – black tea or anything in the shape of a heart*
- *Dark Goddess of the Ninth Heaven – feather or items related to birds*
- *Parvati – lotus flower*
- *Akhilandeshvari – crystals that represent water: aquamarine and blue tourmaline*
- *Beira – pebbles or a hag stone (be careful if shaking stones in the jar!)*
- *Angerona – keys or ribbon to represent her role as the secret keeper*
- *Kerridwen – bay leaf and nutmeg are both connected to the element of fire, and as such transformation and Kerridwen.*

The Spell
Layer your herbs in the jar, three times, so three layers of three. Add any extra items you've selected in the middle layer.
Send your energy and intention clearly into the jar. It may be that you are in need of focus to meet one specific goddess, or you seek blessings for your journey.

Shake your jar each time you feel your mind drifting away, or if a space you are in feels overwhelming to you (you can even carry a little one in your bag for yin moments on the go) – the simple action of shaking the jar stirs up the energy and intention within.

CLOSING YINSIGHTS

The wisdom of darkness and stillness is brought to life by powerful goddess archetypes, representing hope and encouragement. These feminine embodiments can be a much-needed reassurance that you're not alone during the darkest times.

The silence and stillness within the dark can be an opportunity for meditation and reflection, both on one's self and the world. Great transformation can happen in these times of darkness, like in a chrysalis, before something new and beautiful emerges.

When we move through the Wheel of the Year, we cannot progress through the cycle and skip over winter, because we don't fancy the dark and cold. We have to go through the dark to return to the light. The same goes for our shadow selves. We cannot just ignore them on our journey to wholeness – a relatively new term for this is 'spiritual bypassing', which is the use of spiritual ideas and practices to avoid facing unresolved emotional issues and wounds, or difficult emotions and situations.

Working with the dark goddesses and some of the ideas they represent – death, shadow selves, secrets – can be challenging. But it is essential to, in some way, face the darkness in order to create and embrace your whole self. I absolutely understand that you may not be drawn to the dark goddesses in the same way as the golden-haired, maiden beauties of spring and summer. But life, with its yin and yang, is contrast and balance. Just as we need to cast off deeply ingrained ideas of resting being unproductive, because we've been told that our whole lives, I think we also need to cast off these ideas that the crone goddesses with their age and wisdom are not beautiful, or dark goddesses are unappealing or fearsome, or in some way lesser than the young, light beautiful goddess depictions of Aphrodite, Aine, Freya and Ostara. They are all part of one beautiful whole. And if you choose to connect to goddess archetypes, do strive for a balance.

10

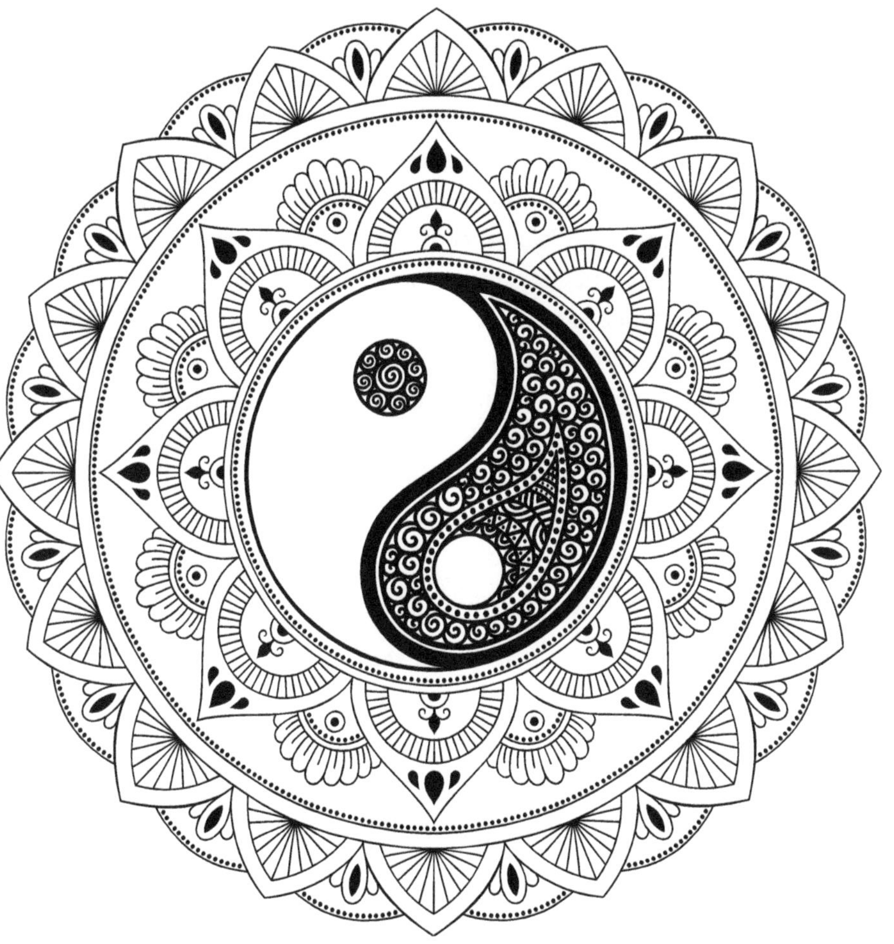

CONCLUSION – GATHERING YIN

In our society, which has made busyness a virtue and has lost itself in the accumulation of power, material things, and continuous growth, many of us find our lives imbalanced and yearn for authenticity, freedom, and simplicity.

Much of our current world and pace of life places the importance of yang over yin. We feel we should always be doing something, and that time not 'doing' is money wasted and opportunities lost. From this, the idea that we can control and master all things is born. An overemphasis of the yang attitude is how we moved from matriarchal societies of support and nurturing to patriarchal societies of domination and control. And frankly, this is partly how we, as a planet and society, have ended up in such a mess, especially when it comes to what we truly value.

A yang society creates anxiety and stress because no one can 'master' life, nature or time. But we rush because society has led us to believe it is possible. What truly nourishes us – yin – is being ignored. We as humans, and indeed all life, should reside in the yin, activating the yang mindfully when needed. We have become a society that is out of balance and full of dis-ease, seeking action and distraction, overthinking, we are easily swayed by trivial concerns such as pettiness, jealousy, cruelty and selfishness…

From verse 28 of the *Tao Te Ching:*[i]

Know the male,
yet keep to the female:
receive the world in your arms.
If you receive the world,
the Tao will never leave you

…

Know the white,
yet keep to the black:
be a pattern for the world.
If you are a pattern for the world,
the Tao will be strong inside you.

i Translation by Stephen Mitchell, 1988.

Yin nourishes all aspects of body and mind and preserves yang. Yin is really the heart of our existence, and yin sees the world as it is, so through this keeping to the yin, you'll receive the world in your arms! We need to take action and reach out at times, but what Lao Tzu and the Taoist tradition say in the Tao Te Ching is that we should be residing in yin as our base point of restfulness and calm, ready to embody yang when we need to. Like our yin tiger, take your time, reside in stillness, so you have the strength to strike your light when needed.

Because of our yin deficiency in the world, we can find it hard to cultivate it, or be unsure how to. Pretending to be okay, that we have it all under control, is a very yang habit – as is feeling that we need to strive, struggle and suffer for our goals, fighting against nature and flow. I'm not saying we shouldn't or don't feel extreme and life-altering grief, pain and loss at times – but prolonged suffering is caused by trying to stuff down these feelings, trying to fight the flow of what is, how we feel and refusing to acknowledge what we need.

This idea of being who we feel we should be, rather than who we are, is, again, trying to battle against nature, our true selves, fighting *wu wei*: it's exhausting!

Yin is the foundation, like the earth: yin creates yang. Doing comes from non-doing. So, we need to nourish yin. Cultivate yin, rest, relaxation and meditation to support health. Lao Tzu, as well as ancient yogis, knew that stillness nourishes action; meditation nourishes the sparks of the mind. Yoga helps us to turn the attention inward, let go of the noise of the outside world and discover pure awareness of the self.

Returning to our true being-ness is to return to wisdom that we already know at our deepest level, but may have forgotten in the noise of everyday life. I know I manage to forget it regularly and I teach yin almost every day! But, as my fellow yogi and friend Michelle once told me, "we teach what we most need to learn."

So, I started this book as part of my own journey, as a teacher of yin yoga looking to dive more deeply into the heritage and roots of yin yoga, uncovering gems of wisdom about yin from Taoism to guide us all on this journey to balance. I have shared here not just *how* to be still, via yoga, spells and meditation, but also, *why* to be still. And how beautiful ideas of astrology, Taoism and seasonal magical work can help us to really *enjoy* a slower way of being in the world.

How can you continue this journey when you put the book down?

How can you move forwards with this idea of yin?

How can you embrace a little yin every day?

How can you quieten the voices that make
you feel guilty when you rest?

As with all things – practice.

- ☾ Enjoy your five-minute spells, but also enjoy ones that unfold over the course of several months.

- ☾ Find little moments of stillness and mindfulness through the day. But slow down for longer whenever you can. Spend whole afternoons or days embracing gentle magic slowly.

- ☾ Enjoy being dynamic but embrace the stillness, knowing that each supports the other in our spiralling whirl of yin and yang, where each side of light and dark contains a little of the opposite as well.

- ☾ Set boundaries: carve out time to explore your path and hold space for yourself.

Seek Space

A line I often use in my yin yoga classes is that "we are on a journey to find space, in our minds but also our bodies". I remind my students that instead of trying to strike a picture-perfect pose, or to stretch ourselves to our very limit, what if we just explored finding a little space?

And here's the thing about space – it's emptiness, it's nothing. And society would have us believe that 'nothing' is a bad thing, a useless thing. But how can we expand if we don't have the space to do so? How can we bring new ideas into a mind that is full? To find space is to find freedom. Space is receptive, just like yin. It is in this yin, feminine, receptive trust we can make space, stillness and freedom. Yin power lies in not forcing, pushing, pulling, but by being and allowing.

Yoga celebrates space, acknowledging the space between thoughts, sensations, elements of our bodies and experiences. By engaging with the expansive fields of sensation and consciousness, working with the body and focused attention, we can harness the power of yoga as this amazing unitive experience.

It is not just our bodies that need space. Give your dreams, emotions and ideas space and time to grow, room to play and change, without expectation of a specific result, or something to 'show' for that time. The space within us and between us is not empty but brimming with information, energy, and connectivity. Space is the master connective tissue, connecting us to, well, everything: to the universal energy, to global cognisance.

Ancient yoga gurus practiced connecting to this space in an extreme manner, separating themselves entirely from the rest of society and meditating in isolated caves and mountains. Their solitary meditations gave them the clarity needed to enlighten their understanding, evaporating the ebb and flow of the never-ending tide of experiences and providing a place from which stillness could flourish.

But we can all find ways to cultivate spaciousness in our bodies, minds and daily lives in smaller ways. We have all most likely at some point found ourselves feeling trapped in lives that did not feel like our own. Maybe you are still there. I want to help, in any small way I can. Just as in yoga class I hold space for my students to be open, present and allowing. I need you, and I implore you, to hold that space for yourself. Loosening your schedule and your consideration of other peoples' ideas, opinions and biases so that you can explore your own. Allow yourself to discover the peacefulness to be found when you stop striving to meet the expectations of society, and instead dare to listen to, and trust in yourself and your own dharma.

Seek Possibility

One of my all-time favourite words is 'possibility'. And it's an amazing feeling when that light of hope and possibility is switched on. Suddenly you can see a path, a way, a choice where before things seemed unknown, scary, or out of reach. I hope that you may, in your journey to stillness, find possibility. Possibility to be who you truly are, without the busyness and constant doing we can get pulled into. Possibility to find clarity, in the effortless action of *wu wei* and to hone where you place your precious attention and love. Possibility of building time to rest and reflect into your regular routine, and release mindless skimming of digital spaces. To release fully, fear that if we were to simply stop, then nothing would get done. On the contrary, time and stillness invite you to reflect and see clearly – where and how to gift your energy... and what to release.

In releasing strict rules, we open ourselves up to possibility. Stillness for a flower that sways in the breeze looks different to the stillness of a rock or pond or a fish. Dare to inquire: what could stillness look like for me? What does stillness from the busyness of my life look like?

Seek *Smarana*

Smarana is a Sanskrit word meaning "remembering what we once knew", and I think it's one of the many reasons why many of us are so excited to connect to the witch archetype, so enchanted with herbs and spices, so delighted to connect to the moon and seasons. It feels more than just interesting: it feels comforting, soothing, and to many, including me, it feels like coming home.

As we dig under the surface of our being, exploring shadow, memory, uncovering and healing we discover what lies deep beneath, our primal way of being in the world, in tune with the world.

Even when I'm not really sure how something works, or what I'm supposed to be doing, connecting to the way of the witch feels like home to me. Weaving together spiritual practice feels like memory.

And I hope it feels comforting to you, too. It is a good reminder that this stuff runs through our bones. So, don't let someone tell you it's pointless or even that it's dangerous. We all may have heard variants of "you should be careful messing with that stuff" or "you don't really believe in that, do you?". To them I say: this is my heritage, don't you dare try and make me fear it, just because it may scare you as an unknown.

And to you I say, keep coming home, my darlings.

Seek Stillness

My wish is that you may find your way to believing in yourself. Believe in yourself enough to trust your body and spirit when they say: *rest.* May you find the space and freedom to focus on what is truly valuable and expend your sacred energy only on what truly matters to you. May you discover your worth without feeling you must constantly prove it with busyness and rushing movement.

May you find within this book ideas that can be a starting point for you to revel in wholehearted presence, harmony in stillness and joyfulness of being.

May you seek and find stillness. May you find rest. May you find magic. May you find your yin and your harmony with nature.

In your stillness, and ongoing journey towards stillness, may you find your bravery, your power, and most of all, your self.

Namaste.

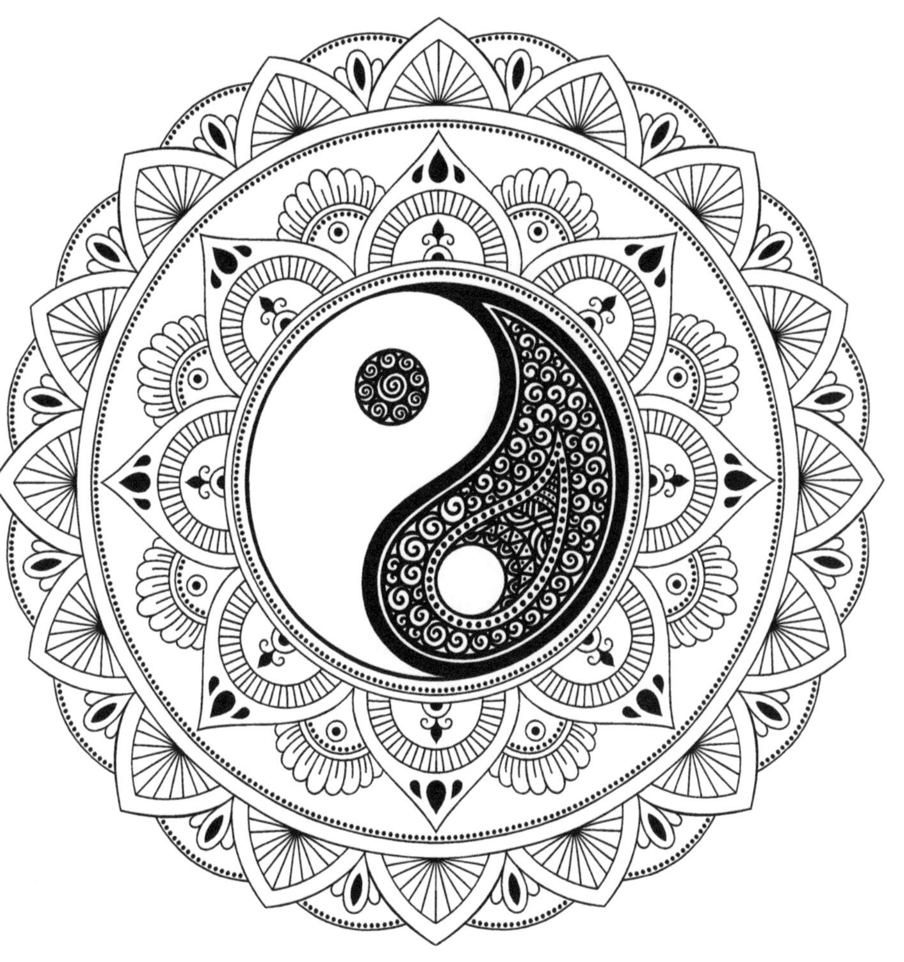

GLOSSARY

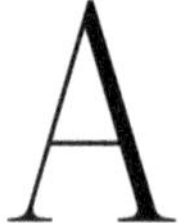

list of words that may be new to you, and their meanings.

Chinese Ideas

Jing

Meaning 'essence' thought to be passed down from ancestors, we are born with a finite amount of ancestral *jing* energy (known as prenatal *jing*) that we consume through life. But we can also acquire *jing* through disciplines such as *qi gong* and meditation and replenish with herbs and nutrition.

Li

A natural order or pattern – like the grain of wood.

Neidan

Inner alchemy in the Taoist tradition.

Qi (pronounced 'chee')

Energy or lifeforce, present in all things and in many forms. In humans *qi* flows through the body in channels known as meridians, connecting all of our major organs.

San Bao – The Three Treasures

Shen: spirit, *jing*: essence, and *qi*: lifeforce together are known as the *san bao* – three treasures – foundations of sustaining human life, each one contributing to overall health and wellbeing of the body.

Shen

This is our spirit or mind, responsible for our consciousness, wisdom, awareness and emotions.

Tao

Literally meaning 'The Way', Tao is perceived as a natural harmonious order underlying all elements of the universe.

Waidan

Outer alchemy in the Taoist tradition.

Wu Wei

Effortless action.

Wu Xing

The Five Phases: *jin* (Metal), *mu* (Wood), *shui* (Water), *huo* (Fire), *tu* (Earth).

Wu Xing is short for *Wu zhong liu xing zhi qi* which translates as; the five types of *qi* dominating at different times. Based on observations of the elements of the natural world, *Wu Xing* is a system used for describing qualities, interactions and relationships.

Yin

Yin is a receptive energy that complements yang's creative energy, making a complete whole. Associated with darkness, stillness and the feminine.

Yang

Yang is an active energy, associated with light and the masculine.

Witchy Words

Witch

The wise one. One who practices magic, which may or may not include practicing spells, divination, charms, rituals and ceremonies. Various etymological roots include the old English words *wicca* and *wicche* meaning wise and *weik* meaning to bend and wind.

Green Witch

A witch whose practice focuses on nature, natural materials and energies. Green Witches are often skilled herbalists, gardeners and wildcrafters. Green Witches attune to the cycles of nature and see natural places as sacred.

Hedge Witch

A Hedge Witch is a witch who has knowledge and skills about herbs as well as astral projection and divination. She acts as an intermediary between the spirit or astral realms and the material realm.

Kitchen Witch

A Kitchen Witch or Hearth Witch focuses their magical practice on the home and hearth. Kitchen Witchery often involves the use of essential oils, herbs, foods and everyday objects.

Yoga Witch

I'm certainly not the first to blend these two elements together. Look up #YogaWitch on Instagram and you'll find over thirty thousand images! But I am honoured to have done my part to cultivate the idea of the Yoga Witch: one who weaves wisdom, practice, and holds space for others on their yoga journey.

Paganism

An umbrella term covering a wide range of beliefs, it can be applied to many non-mainstream religions. The word pagan is often used to describe any earth-based spirituality.

Altar

A space used as the focus for ritual, especially for making offerings to a deity and working with spells.

Alchemy

A process of transformation and/or creation. Ancient forerunner of chemistry, alchemy is the means of taking the ordinary and turning it into something extraordinary, sometimes in ways that cannot be explained by traditional science.

Cauldron

The cauldron is a symbol of transformation and rebirth. Cauldrons can represent the female aspect of divinity, the womb.

Correspondence

Charts of symbolic connections in the natural and magical world, tables of correspondence help us connect and group together elements for spell and ritual work. For example, the moon corresponds to colours of silver and white. You can use existing correspondence from books or work to create your own.

Manifestation

This is the writing down or focusing on what you want to bring into your life. One may perform a manifestation spell, ritual, meditation, or create manifestation bottles, boxes and bowls.

Sigils

A sigil is a picture that represents a desire or intention. They are most commonly created by writing out the intention, then condensing the letters down to form an icon.

Spell

A spell is an intentional focusing of energy to achieve an objective. Spells are traditionally written or spoken, the power of words and intention being vital. Spellcraft is the craft of making spells.

Sympathetic Magic

Sympathetic magic is a type of magic based on imitation or connection.

Witches Ladder

A spell consisting of tying nine knots in a length of rope or ribbon to 'bind' energy within the item. Artwork and writings from fifteenth and sixteenth century Europe depict witches selling wind to sailors using this means! The sailors would buy witches ladders bound within the energy of the wind and storms for use at sea (there is an image of one such transaction at the Witchcraft and Magic Museum at Boscastle, classified under Sea Witchcraft).

Yoga Words

Asana

Physical posture of yoga. Translated, it means 'seat' because that's where is all began; before fancy balances and elaborate poses. The connection of yoga was found in a simple seated pose.

Ayurveda

The 'science of life', considered the sister science of yoga that utilises movement, meditation and diet for holistic wellbeing.

Dharma

Our natures' true calling and the path to refine our Buddha within.

Dosha

Based in the theory of five basic elements found in the universe: space, air, fire, water and earth. These combine to form three bodily energies, called *doshas*, in Ayurveda. They are *Vata dosha* (space and air); *Pitta dosha* (fire and water); and *Kapha dosha* (water and earth).

Mantra

A sound or chant often used in meditation. A mantra can focus concentration on one purpose and help still the mind.

Namaste
A classic greeting and parting phrase for yogis and Hindus, with many translations around honouring to one another, my favourite is "the light in me honours the light in you".

Prana
Life force, vital energy.

Pranayama
Exercises in yoga using the breath to direct and expand the flow of *prana* (energy) in our bodies.

Sanskrit
Ancient Indian language thought to have inherent power.

Siddhis
Attainment, fulfilment and/or power.

Smarana
'Remembering' or 'uncovering'.

Yin Yoga
Yin yoga works deep into connective tissues of the body with long held stretches. The postures work into the energy flows, or meridians, of the body. While passive, yin yoga challenges you to find peace in poses for three to five minutes (sometimes longer).

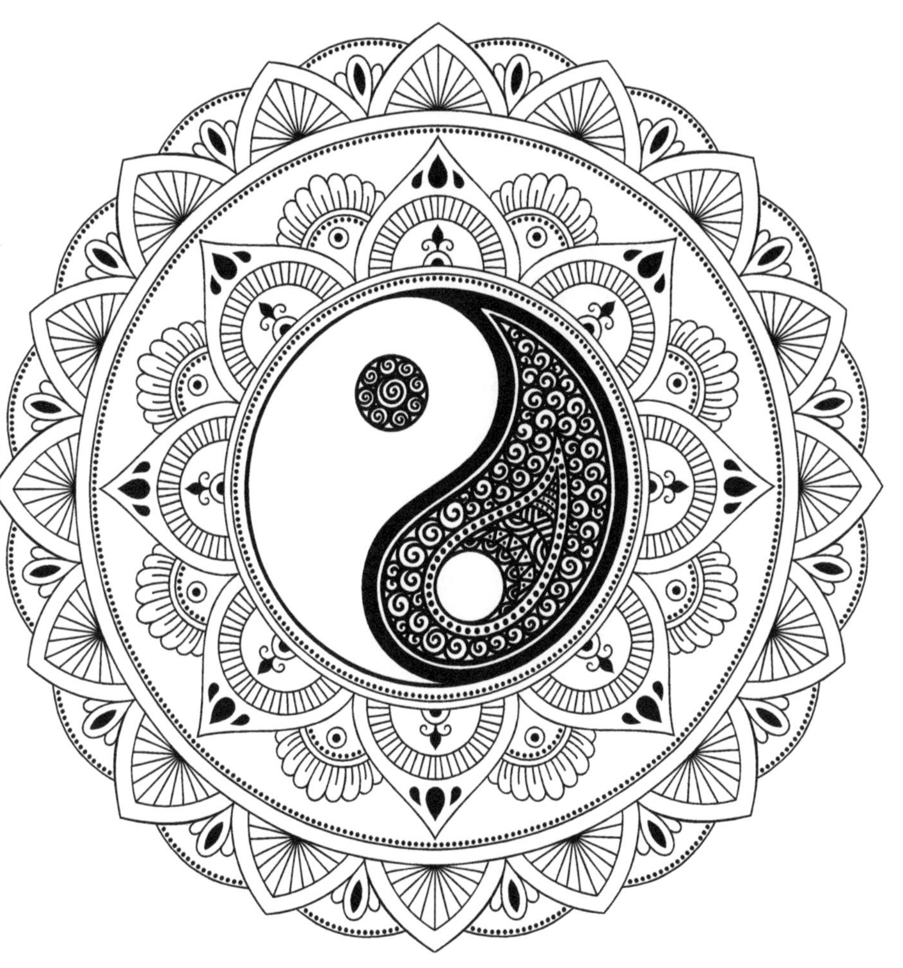

READING LIST

More on Yin Yoga

The Complete Guide to Yin Yoga – Bernie Clarke

Brightening Our Inner Skies – Norman Blair

Yin Yoga – Paul Grilley

Insight Yoga – Sarah Powers

Yoga: The Spirit and Practice of Moving Into Stillness – Erich Schiffmann

On Witches and Cauldrons

The Witch's Cauldron: The Craft, Lore and Magick of Ritual Vessels – Laura Tempest Zakroff

On Dark Goddesses

Dancing in the Flames: The Dark Goddess of Transformation and Consciousness – Marion Woodman and Elinor Dickson

Medicine and Finding Balance

Medicine Woman: Reclaiming the Soul of Healing – Lucy H. Pearce

The Yin and Yang of Self-Compassion: Cultivating Kindness and Strength in the Face of Difficulty – Kristin Neff

The Yellow Emperor's Classic of Medicine translated – Maoshing Ni

Basic Theories of Traditional Chinese Medicine – Zhu Bing and Wang Hongcai

Tao and Finding Stillness

The Tao Te Ching
One of the texts that started it all…just like Patanjali's *Yoga Sutras* for yoga. Written by Lao Tzu more than two thousand years ago, intended as a guide to cultivating a life of peace, serenity, compassion and harmony with the lifeforce of the universe. These are two translations that are available freely online:

Translation by Gia-fu feng and Jane English: terebess.hu/english/tao/gia.html#1972

You can also see a version at taoism.net:
The Tao of Craft: Fu Talismans and Casting Sigils in the Eastern Esoteric Tradition – Benebell Wen

Cultivating Stillness: Taoist Manual for Transforming Body and Mind – Eva Wong

Taoism: An Essential Guide – Eva Wong

Complete I Ching: The Definitive Translation – Taoist Master Alfred Huang

Tao: The Watercourse Way – Alan Watts

And of course:
The Tao of Pooh – Benjamin Hoff. Those who read my book, *Yoga for Witches*, will know that my very first yoga book was called *The Beginner Bear's Book of Yoga*, so I am all about utilising bears to explain spiritual topics!

On Alchemy and the Psyche

Psychology and Alchemy: The Collected Works of C. G. Jung

The Alchemy of Menopause – Cathy Skipper

The Modern Alchemist: A Guide to Personal Transformation – Richard Miller and Iona Miller

Online Resources

Tao, Sigils and Chinese Culture

benebellwen.com

About Yin Yoga, and Pioneers of the Practice

yinyoga.com
yogawithnorman.co.uk
sarahpowers.com
paulgrilley.com

Moon Lore

chaninicholas.com
yasminboland.com

Compassion

Both websites share a wealth of studies into the benefits of self-compassion, meditation and mindfulness

compassioninstitute.com
self-compassion.org

Meditations with me!

A great free resource and over sixty of my own meditations to help you journey to stillness.

insig.ht/sentiayoga

ABOUT THE AUTHOR

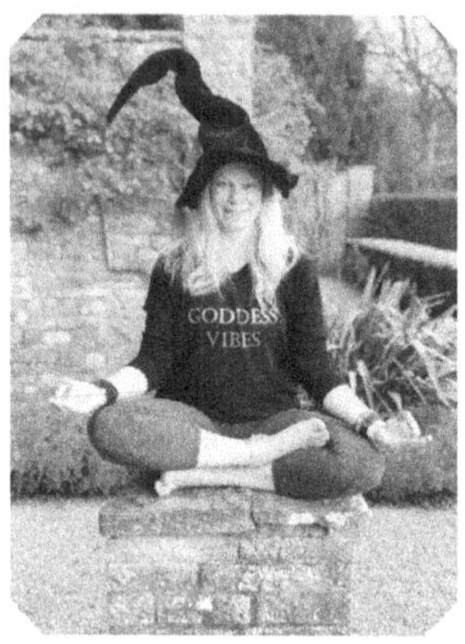

Sarah is a yoga and meditation teacher based in Bath, UK (once named after a goddess: the ancient roman town of Aquae Sulis). Her background is in science: she holds an MSc in Psychology and Neuroscience and has studied at Bath, Exeter and Harvard universities.

Sarah has practiced yoga since the age of seven. Weaving in her love of all things myth, magic and goddess, Sarah is passionate about creating practices to inspire and transform. Through yoga, meditation and ritual she aims to help everyone connect to their own special magic and inner power.

ABOUT THE ARTIST

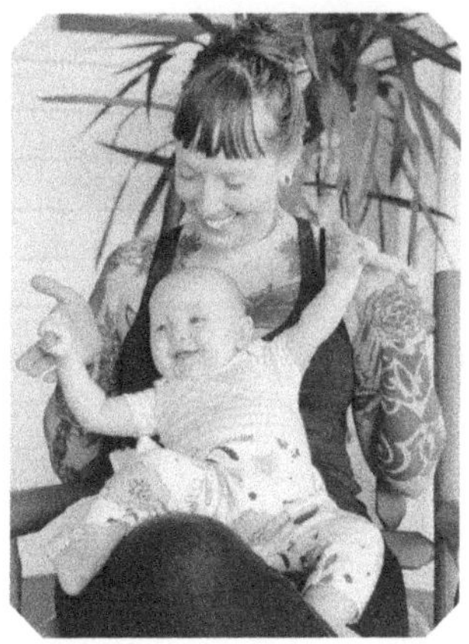

Hannah Dansie's work draws from influences derived from iconoclasm, mythology, and the natural environment. Using familiar imagery and symbolism her images try to illustrate the connections that go unseen between ourselves and the natural world, while creating a sense of nostalgia for the dreamlike world of fairytales and folklore. All works are created in acrylic, ink, and gouache.

Hannah was born and raised near the redwoods and beaches of Northern California. She studied fine art at Central Saint Martin's University in London, England, where she graduated with a BFA Honors degree in 2004. She works and resides in Madison County, NC with her loving husband and daughter. Her work has been shown in Asheville at The Satellite Gallery, The Center for Visual Artists in Greensboro NC, The Red Truck Gallery in New Orleans LA, The Convent Philly in Philadelphia PA, and The Gristle Gallery in Brooklyn NY. You can find a large collection of her prints and originals on permanent display at The Horse and Hero in Asheville, NC.

hannah-dansie.com
instagram.com/hannahdansie
facebook.com/HannahDansie.Art

ABOUT WOMANCRAFT

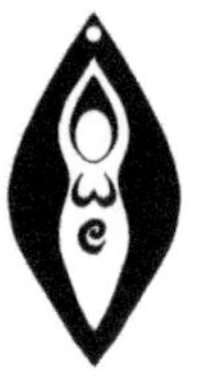

Womancraft Publishing was founded on the revolutionary vision that women and words can change the world. We act as midwife to transformational women's words that have the power to challenge, inspire, heal and speak to the silenced aspects of ourselves.

We believe that:

- ☾ books are a fabulous way of transmitting powerful transformation,
- ☾ values should be juicy actions, lived out,
- ☾ ethical business is a key way to contribute to conscious change.

At the heart of our Womancraft philosophy is fairness and integrity. Creatives and women have always been underpaid. Not on our watch! We split royalties 50:50 with our authors. We work on a full circle model of giving and receiving: reaching backwards, supporting TreeSisters' reforestation projects, and forwards via Worldreader, providing books at no cost to education projects for girls and women.

We are proud that Womancraft is walking its talk and engaging so many women each year via our books and online. Join the revolution! Sign up to the mailing list at womancraftpublishing.com and find us on social media for exclusive offers:

womancraftpublishing

womancraftbooks

womancraft_publishing

Signed copies of all titles available from shop.womancraftpublishing.com

USE OF WOMANCRAFT WORK

Often women contact us asking if and how they may use our work. We love seeing our work out in the world. We love you sharing our words further. And we ask that you respect our hard work by acknowledging the source of the words.

We are delighted for short quotes from our books – up to 200 words – to be shared as memes or in your own articles or books, provided they are clearly accompanied by the author's name and the book's title.

We are also very happy for the materials in our books to be shared amongst women's communities: to be studied by book groups, discussed in classes, read from in ceremony, quoted on social media… with the following provisos:

- If content from the book is shared in written or spoken form, the book's author and title must be referenced clearly.
- The only person fully qualified to teach the material from any of our titles is the author of the book itself. There are no accredited teachers of this work. Please do not make claims of this sort.
- If you are creating a course devoted to the content of one of our books, its title and author must be clearly acknowledged on all promotional material (posters, websites, social media posts).
- The book's cover may be used in promotional materials or social media posts. The cover art is copyright of the artist and has been licensed exclusively for this book. Any element of the book's cover or font may not be used in branding your own marketing materials when teaching the content of the book, or content very similar to the original book.
- No more than two double page spreads, or four single pages of any book may be photocopied as teaching materials.

We are delighted to offer a 20% discount of over five copies going to one address. You can order these on our webshop, or email us. If you require further clarification, email us at:

info@womancraftpublishing.com

ALSO FROM
WOMANCRAFT PUBLISHING

YOGA
for
WITCHES

SARAH ROBINSON

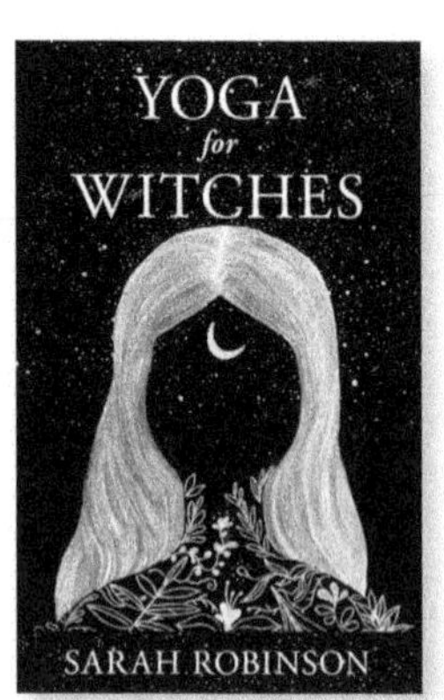

Yoga for Witches explores a new kind of journey, connecting two powerful spiritual disciplines, with enchanting effects! Witchcraft and yoga share many similarities that are explored in combination, in this groundbreaking new title from Sarah Robinson, certified yoga instructor and experienced witch.

Yoga for Witches shares exercises, poses and the knowledge you need to connect to your own special magic and inner power.

☾ Explore how ancient yogis sought out magic.

☾ Weave magic through spells, mantra, meditation and yoga practice.

☾ Discover some of the goddesses and gods of yogic and witch culture.

☾ Connect to the power of the sun, moon and earth via witchcraft and yoga.

☾ Explore the magic of the chakras.

Wild & Wise: sacred feminine meditations for women's circles and personal awakening

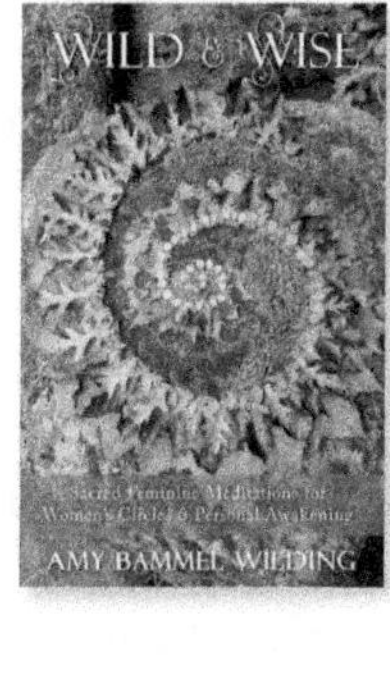

Amy Wilding

The stunning debut by Amy Wilding is not merely a collection of guided meditations, but a potent tool for personal and global transformation. The meditations beckon you to explore the powerful realm of symbolism and archetypes, inviting you to access your wild and wise inner knowing.
Suitable for reflective reading or to facilitate healing and empowerment for women who gather in red tents, moon lodges, women's circles and ceremonies.

This rich resource is an answer to "what can we do to go deeper?" that many in circles want to know.

Jean Shinoda Bolen, MD

Sisters of the Solstice Moon (Book 1 of the When She Wakes series)

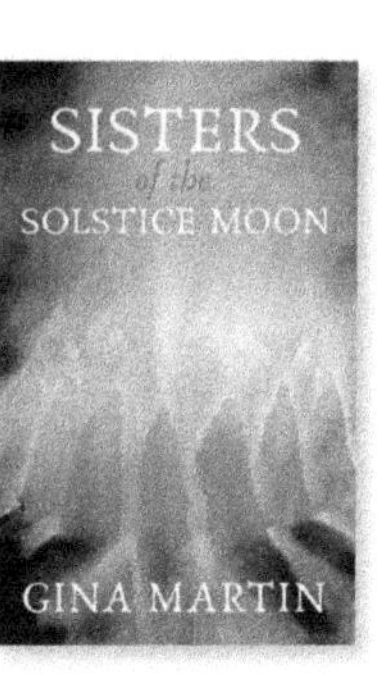

Gina Martin

On the Winter Solstice, thirteen women across the world see the same terrifying vision. Their world is about to experience ravaging destruction. All that is now sacred will be destroyed. Each answers the call, to journey to Egypt, and save the wisdom of the Goddess.

An imagining…or is it a remembering…of the end of matriarchy and the emergence of global patriarchy, this book brings alive long dead cultures from around the world and brings us closer to the lost wisdoms that we know in our bones.

Moon Time: harness the ever-changing energy of your menstrual cycle

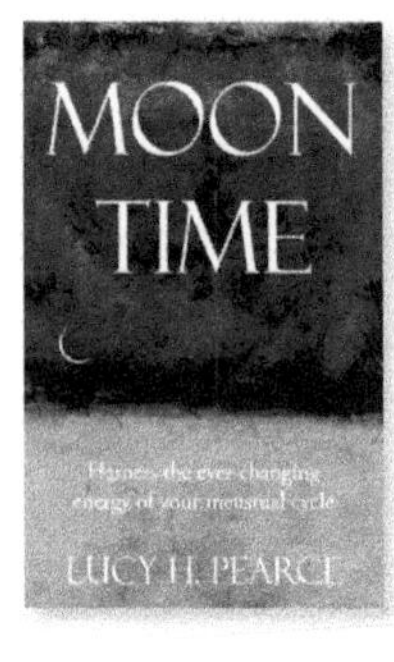

Lucy H. Pearce

Hailed as 'life-changing' by women around the world, *Moon Time* shares a fully embodied understanding of the menstrual cycle. Full of practical insight, empowering resources, creative activities and passion, this book will put women back in touch with their body's wisdom.

This book is a wonderful journey of discovery. Lucy not only guides us through the wisdom inherent in our wombs, our cycles and our hearts, but also encourages us to share, express, celebrate and enjoy what it means to be female! A beautiful and inspiring book full of practical information and ideas.

Miranda Gray, author of *Red Moon* and *The Optimized Woman*

Medicine Woman: reclaiming the soul of healing

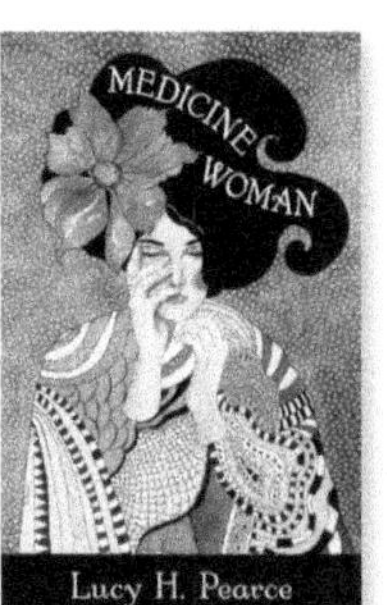

Lucy H. Pearce

Nautilus Silver Award 2018

This audacious questioning of the current medical system's ability to deal with the modern epidemic of chronic illness, combines a raw personal memoir of sickness and healing, woven through with voices of dozens of other long-term sick women of the world and a feminine cultural critique that digs deep into the roots of patriarchal medicine. *Medicine Woman* voices a deep yearning for a broader vision of what it means to be human than our current paradigm allows for, calling on an ancient archetype of healing, Medicine Woman, to re-vision how we can navigate sickness and harness its transformational powers in order to heal.

Packed with dozens of healing arts exercises and hundreds of medicine questions to help integrate body and mind in the healing process.

Lightning Source UK Ltd.
Milton Keynes UK
UKHW012129291021
393062UK00003B/879